Stroke After Stroke:

A Rower's Pilgrimage

by

Barbara Polan

To Amy and the rest of the

online Stroke Tribe

Always remember, there's more to life than rowing - but not much.

-- Donald Beer (former Olympian sculler) to John Biglow (Olympic hopeful)
in *The Amateurs: The Story of Four Young Men and Their Quest for an Olympic Gold Medal*,
by David Halberstam

Table Of Contents

Preface

This book is intended for survivors of stroke and everyone else facing a return to life devastated by any disability. It might be of interest even to people who have no expectation of ever becoming disabled. I hope my contribution to the stroke recovery conversation will be to inspire survivors to persevere and to thoughtfully explore some of the facets of recovery - the physical and emotional challenges that inevitably follow. I would like to help survivors understand disability and put it into the proper context of their lives.

As a stroke survivor (struck Nov. 12, 2009, at the age of 52), I find my most difficult non-physical challenge since then to be re-defining and understanding my expectations and goals. I have always been a goal-oriented person, someone propelled along to a well-designed endpoint. For 50 years, reaching the destination was more satisfying to me than the trek. Pre-stroke, there were many times I tried to savor the moment, but, honestly, it came across to me as inefficient, a waste of time even.

In my quest for recovery, I have found other survivors - for equal parts understanding, camaraderie, comfort, information, encouragement and insight. Please note that I am not an expert and I have no medical background. Think of me, instead, as a friend traveling along a similar path.

The following books written by stroke survivors may be considered required reading for stroke survivors:

Never Give Up: My Stroke, My Recovery and My Return to the NFL, by Tedy Bruschi, a New

England Patriots linebacker at the time of his stroke.

My Stroke of Insight, by Jill Bolt Taylor, a neuroscientist.

Don't Leave Me This Way: or when I get back on my feet you'll be sorry, by Julia Fox Garrison.

The Tales of a Stroke Patient, by Joyce Hoffman.

My Last Degree: A Therapist Goes Home After Stroke, by Rebecca Dutton, a physical therapist.

In addition, there is one written by a stroke rehab expert, not a survivor, who is considered by survivors to be the person most knowledgeable about stroke and stroke recovery: *Stronger After Stroke*, by Peter Levine.

During my recovery from an ischemic stroke caused by the dissection of my right carotid artery, I've kept a blog (at barbpolansrecovery.blogspot.com) about my recovery, which constitutes a large part of this narrative. I have left my blog entries as-is; any changes (notes, corrections, etc.) I've made in this account of my journey are within square brackets.

Although it might not be the experience of every stroke survivor, I have found stroke recovery to be as much an emotional and philosophical journey as a physical one.

I see now that in some ways I was atypical of a stroke survivor:

1. I was 52 years old at the time, relatively "young" to have a stroke.

2. I was the most fit I'd been in my life: I had recently given up a daily three-mile run for rowing a gig boat

in Gloucester Harbor, near where I live. I was at a healthy weight.

3. I had low total cholesterol, and my slightly high blood pressure was well controlled by a beta-blocker.

4. I had a demanding full-time job in a profession I adored.

In other ways I was typical:

1. I was female.

2. My children were adults

3. I thought I was safe from certain health issues. I knew, given that both my maternal grandmother and my mother died as the result of colon cancer, that was my most likely exit, and I was diligent about having colonoscopies. Given my physical condition and medical history, in my mind stroke was out of the realm of the possible.

And, most typically:

4. I expected tomorrow to be like today.

Pre-Stroke

The Day minus 7 months

We live in a loosely knit neighborhood in Gloucester, Massachusetts; we have periodic neighborhood celebrations, and the women have formed a book group.

At a Thanksgiving 2008 party, our next-door neighbor tried to convince my husband, Tom, to join him in participating in the upcoming first Gloucester Triathlon. Tom was hesitant – although he had recently given up playing hockey four times a week and the idea of getting in shape for the triathlon appealed to him, he wasn't sure he could commit the time – he had a one-hour commute and long hours of work at a start-up. Another neighbor suggested that he join the local rowing club; its members rowed pilot gig boats in Gloucester Harbor. It was a hard workout and relaxing to be out on the harbor, he said.

While I encouraged Tom to prepare for the triathlon, I idly thought about joining the rowing club myself. Running had become stale: I had plateaued at three miles, and I could use a change - rowing pilot gig boats might be it.

History of pilot gig boats

While pilot gig boats are currently used for recreation – often racing – they were originally built in Cornwall, England, as working boats. At times since then, they have served as rescue boats for the crews of foundering ships, dashing out to haul shipwreck survivors out of the water.

The pilot gig's primary function, though, and the reason for its unique design and its name is to ferry a local "pilot" out to an incoming merchant ship. As a ship bearing items obtained in distant lands sailed into a harbor, competing pilot gig boats raced to greet the vessel, with the first one to the ship rewarded by having the opportunity to provide a pilot to show the vessel a safe way through the harbor and to a land-based merchant interested in purchasing the goods. The pilot and his crew would then be paid a cut of the products changing hands.

With ferrying the pilot as its purpose, a gig boat, even though it is built of wood and quite heavy, is streamlined for speed and has eight stationary seats: one in the stern for a coxswain (cox) who steers and directs the rowers, six for rowers to power out to the ship, and one in the bow for the pilot.

At the time I had the stroke, the Gloucester Gig Rowing Club had two pilot gig boats, which were used daily for recreation from May into November in Gloucester Harbor. The rowers also participated in races against other gigs and some whaleboats along the New England coast.

On a perfect row, the sun would set over West Gloucester as we passed Ten-Pound Island, on the east side of the harbor. The surface of the water would ripple like quicksilver and dazzle us with hundreds – maybe thousands - of orange diamonds from the sunset.

The Day minus 12 days

After six months of rowing in the Gloucester Gig Rowing Club, I started participating in races.

That October, I was signed up to go to the annual "Head of the Weir" race in Hull on Halloween 2009. It is a four- or five-mile race, and preparation included challenging daily one-hour practices with the other team members, designed to get us used to rowing with each other and being instructed by the cox.

On one practice for the "Weir," there were six of my favorite rowers (actually five rowers who all love a significant workout and a wonderful cox) in my preferred boat, the Siren Song. We rowed hard for 20 minutes, keeping our oars in perfect synch, and then took a water break, propping the butts of the oars under a wooden strip that runs the length of the boat.

Each of the Siren Song's oars is a 15-foot solid piece of ash, with exposed wood on the shaft and painted red blades trimmed in white. Where the oar sits on the gunwale, between two pegs, called tholepins, there is a 15-inch band of leather to protect the oar from being worn by the gunwale.

Throughout the row, I tried for perfect form: keeping my limbs, back, eyes and oar all in their correct positions. To row, I leaned forward and dipped the blade into the water so that its top edge was just below the surface; then I leaned back, pushing back with my legs, pulling with my arms. Perfect.

I was sitting on the port side of the gig, my right hip up against the gunwale, with the blade of my oar out the starboard side, so the butt of the oar swung to the left of my body as I got to the end of each stroke. The leather sleeve on the shaft pivoted back and forth between the two pins, hitting the pins at both ends of each stroke, rhythmically banging: thunk, pause, thunk, pause, six oars in unison. We were a perfect team in harmony.

After most of our one-hour practice, the cox turned us back to the dock and called for power strokes (as hard as we could pull) for the final 20 minutes. I did my best to keep in time with the rower in seat 6, called the "stroke," and pulled as powerfully as I could. Then my oar "crabbed" (also called "caught a crab.")

13

"Crabbing" is the name for an oar getting caught by the water, which twists the oar blade and makes it nearly impossible to control. My oar had crabbed on several previous rows, and I knew the recovery procedure: raise the end that's in my hands over my head and wait for the pull of the water to subside, then lever the blade out of the water, and start again, catching up with the other rowers.

During this practice, though, I forgot the remedy and struggled, but failed, to control my oar. With the water forcing its will on the blade end, I pulled against it in an attempt to wrestle the blade out of the water and resume rowing.

In the battle, the fore tholepin, a one-and-a half-inch in diameter dowel-like piece of oak, acted as the pivot point of a lever and could not handle the pressure. It broke – actually ripped – in two. The cox stopped the boat, and one of the other rowers offered me one of his pins so that the row could resume; he evidently knew how to row using just one pin, a skill that surprised me. The rest of the row was uneventful, and the following day when I arrived for practice, a new pin was in place.

The Day minus 10 days

The start of the "Head of the Weir" race in Hull on October 31, 2009 (the date is easy to remember because some light-hearted rowers in another boat were in Viking costumes and even our serious Siren Song had a skull attached to her bow), was in a salt marsh with very smooth water. It was exceptionally windy that day, though, which produces waves in less protected water, and the racecourse included a channel with a strong tidal current.

Together, those factors promised to make the race challenging – once we got out of the salt marsh and into the rough water, the size of the waves meant we were pulling our oar blades through water only about half the time, and air the other half; as hard as we could in the former, then with our oars set free in the latter, very choppy and uneven stroking. At one point, despite rowing our hardest, we were stationary compared to the shore. We later described it as being in a vortex.

Facing the stern, the rowers watched boat after boat (and most of the kayaks) head for the shore, fleeing for safety. I would occasionally turn my head the opposite direction to check out just how foul the conditions were, and every time, a wave smashed into my face, so I stopped turning my head. Eventually the chase boat, a motorboat following the racers and responsible for helping rowers in trouble, was bobbing just behind us; I was insulted. As soon as I thought, "We don't need no stinking chase boat," a kayak next to us flipped. Our cox looked her way, as though considering whether we should retrieve her, but the chase boat materialized next to her, so we continued on.

At one point while we were flailing, I thought that this race was not what I had expected and promised myself – presciently, it may turn out – that I would never, ever be crazy enough to race in it again. It was taking everything I had in me – every muscle, every effort, every bit of determination. Even our very experienced cox was baffled about what the best route along the course was.

Once we rounded a point and were headed directly to the beach that was the finish line, we knew we had made it and plowed ahead, riding a wave onto the sand.

As a wooden boat, the Siren Song is heavy, but empty, can be lifted and carried by several rowers. That day, because of the water she was carrying, it took rowers packed along each side to move her to the trailer. Once

15

our team was gathered on shore, our cox pulled off his rubber boots and poured at least a gallon of water out of each.

Giddy with relief, we headed to the Hull Lifesaving Museum, where rowers were gathering out of the wind. We, of course, had brought beer. I, of course, was the one who was chastised by one of the host rowers for drinking in a public place. Somehow, I am frequently – and usually inaccurately - labeled an instigator. Later, in the rehab hospital, I was labeled "impulsive" because of my tendency to ignore rules, but I think I was being blamed for things I didn't do.

"Where are you from?" the accusing rower asked. "Don't you know about the Massachusetts open container law?"

"Not a problem," I responded, and then turned away from him to fetch a Styrofoam cup. Most of the other teams' rowers were drinking coffee in Styrofoam cups to warm up; once the head of my beer subsided, I blended right in. I wondered how coffee could suffice for the others after such a terrifying row.

Before the medals were awarded, one of the organizers announced that out of more than 100 boats that had started, only 42 had finished. Who cared that we had come in seventh out of seven gig boats? What mattered was that we had come in at all – that we had not given up.

The Day minus 4 days

My next – and what ended up as my last before the stroke – race was the following weekend, and the competition was billed by the club in Plymouth that had organized it as the "Northeast Rowing Championship" races. For this event, our club had decided to enter both the men's and the women's (instead of mixed gender) gig boat races. I was on our women's team in the Siren Song, in a race that included five other gig boats, including a couple made of fiberglass. Traditional pilot gig boats are made of wood, but among the nearby clubs that focus more on competition than on recreation or tradition, there has been a recent trend toward fiberglass, which makes their boats significantly lighter and faster than the wooden boats. With just our two wooden boats, our club was used to coming in last in races.

In fact, the men's race was right before ours, and our men's team – in the Siren Song – remained in last place, out of six boats, throughout the race, including the finish.

When time for the women's race came around, we took our places in the gig and rowed to the starting line, an imaginary line from a buoy to a marker on the shore. Five other boats joined us, roughly lined up side-by-side. One by one, the man in control of starting and timing the race OK'd our positions, bows lined up. We, the farthest from the starter, were the first approved. But, as the starter continued along the line and told the other boats how to adjust their positions, we drifted from ours. In an attempt to correct our position, our cox had us make a small loop to get our angle straight. With our stern at the starting line – that is, completely turned backwards – the sixth boat was approved, and the starting horn blasted.

There we were, in our big ol' wooden Siren Song, starting both stern-forward and in sixth place.

I tried to hide my dismay. "We can do this," I shouted.

"Power strokes until I tell you to stop," our cox called out after she had our boat pivoted and pointing bow first.

Power strokes it was, all of us pulling as hard as we could. Personally, I was fueled by the adrenaline rush of the unfairness of the start. We sprinted, as only a wooden gig can – slogging along like a tub. But it was fast enough to pass the boat in fifth place while we were on the first leg (about one mile long in a triangular course). With rowers' backs toward the bow of the boat, rowers don't see a boat they're overtaking until they're already side-by-side; then the passing rowers watch the fallen faces of the rowers in the flagging boat.

I tried not to think of the five other boats ahead. An experienced rower in our club once told me during a race that "We're only ever racing against one boat – the one right in front of us."

We were on the longest leg of the race – a three-mile straight stretch – and still sprinting. At times, between our own exhortations to each other, we could hear the shouts of our comrades on shore. We kept it up around the turn to the last leg - passing Grace, from Belfast, Maine, as we powered on - and then all the way to the end.

As we crossed the finish line in fourth place, we were exhausted, but proud anyway, and still irked that the start had been fouled up. As we climbed out of the Siren Song to congratulations on a race well rowed, the timer approached and told us he'd seen that he had blown the horn too early, and had timed how long it had taken for us to return to the starting line, then removed that from our final time, which placed us third, behind two fiberglass boats.

It had been a one-hour flat-out sprint, and we had done well.

After the race, Tom and I drove to a nearby town to visit and stay overnight (a Saturday) with friends. While there, I had too many glasses of wine. At the end of the evening, Tom accompanied me up the stairs, but I stumbled along the way, and my speech was slurred; all of

18

us blamed the alcohol. The next morning (Sunday), I felt fine, and Tom and I went home to Gloucester.

The Day minus 3 days

On Monday, I woke up at home with a swollen and puffy red right eye, with no pain. I jumped to the conclusion it was conjunctivitis, despite no gunk oozing from it, then called my doctor's office and asked to be seen. In the office, the LPN checked my eye and determined it was *not* conjunctivitis, just swelling around the eye that did not involve the eyeball. She concluded it was caused by an allergy, which sounded wrong to me.

"But I'm not allergic to anything," I objected.

"A new soap or moisturizer?" she asked, then ignored my shaking head.

The Day minus 2 days

I worked at home all day Tuesday preparing for a consultant who would be meeting with me and with my employer's sales reps in two days. The consultant was very expensive, and I planned to get every dollar's worth. At the time, I was the general manager of a small community newspaper based in Westborough, Mass.

The Day minus 1 day

Ditto ... nothing out of the ordinary. I rowed twice that day – a recreational row in the morning and a conditioning row at 3 p.m.

The Stroke — "The Day"

Later, I started a blog. I wrote this entry six weeks after that:

On Nov. 12, 2009, I woke up and got ready for work as usual. Nothing was amiss until I got downstairs and tried to walk across the kitchen to where Tom was standing; at that point, my left ankle started collapsing when I stepped on my left foot, so that I was dragging my left foot across the linoleum floor. I was wearing Dansko clogs, in which I sometimes roll my ankles, so I dismissed the problem. I got my make-up bag out of my purse and immediately dropped it on the floor. When I picked it up, it immediately dropped to the floor again.

"What's wrong?" Tom asked.

"Nothing." I definitely considered nothing wrong.

I picked up the bag for the third time and dragged me and my left foot to the half-bath near the kitchen, where I applied my make-up. Those of you who know me ... know that the make-up application could not have taken more than two minutes. At the end, I straightened up and fell over to my left, knocking my head into the window trim and knocking the toilet paper roll onto the floor; the toilet paper holder in that bathroom is just a bar that curves from against the wall forward to create a place to slip on the roll; it's the toilet paper holder that is absolutely the easiest onto which to replace an expired roll - no excuses for leaving the next user without paper, one of my pet peeves.

At the sound of my fall (or was it the very loud, "Shit! Shit! Shit! Shit! Shit! Shit! Shit!" that followed that tumble?), Tom appeared at the bathroom door and asked if I was okay.

"Yes, but can you please put the roll back on the holder?"

"No," he said. "I want to see what's wrong with you."

"Nothing's wrong with me. I'm just having a little trouble with my ankle. Do me a favor, please, and put the roll on, okay?

"No, we have a bigger problem than the roll not being there."

"What do you mean? What if someone uses the toilet and there's no paper here? I hate that. It's a simple request - can't you just put the roll on?"

Now I was getting mad.

Tom straightened me up, one hand on each of my arms, just below the shoulders and he peered into my face, looking for something. I was baffled.

"There's something terribly wrong, Barb - the left side of your body is not working. Smile at me." I did, even though I was still irked that he wouldn't replace the roll.

"Something is definitely wrong," he said. "The left side of your face isn't working right either."

How can a face not "work right?"

"I'm fine," I insisted. "Can you please put the roll on before I head for work?"

"You're not going to work today - you've had a stroke. You're not going anywhere except the emergency room."

That was not an option ... I am as reliable as the sun [trite metaphor], which is why I had, over the 11 years I'd worked at the paper, gone from being a reporter to being general manager. Although I often telecommuted, not going to work on a day I was supposed to be in the office was not ever an option. I didn't miss a day, ever.

In fact, before that day, I'd had a perfect life and I was very grateful for it: a wonderful, interesting husband and two grown children (at the time, our son was married, living on Long Island and running his own business, which he loved - and our daughter was a senior - a music major - at Columbia University; we lived in a lovely old historic house in Gloucester, a house that requires endless improvements, but is well worth the effort – with a stucco exterior, slate roof, beautiful yard with granite outcroppings and a view of the sea. And it has a name -- Bayberry Ledge...

Tom got me to the ER after all, by lying and promising to drive me to work (to get me into the passenger seat of the car). I let him because my commute is more than an hour and my car is a standard, so I wasn't sure my left leg was going to be able to push in the clutch. After the ER at Addison-Gilbert in Gloucester, I was transferred to Massachusetts General Hospital for two days, and then to Spaulding Rehab-Boston for four weeks. While there, I learned more about my condition and how to walk with a quad-cane (a cane with four feet). I also learned what compassionate, supportive friends and family I have – they all stepped up to help me through the ordeal.

One strong cheerleader my boss, encourages me to identify progress every single day, which now, six weeks later, is sometimes a challenge.

My niece Emily gave me the book Julie and Julia, by Julie Powell, that Christmas, and when I finished it, I thought that since starting a blog when she took on the challenge of working through every recipe in Julia Child's Mastering the Art of French Cooking was such a good idea for Julie, it could also work for me as a way to look back and see progress during my recovery journey - no less daunting, I think, than mastering French cooking.

Stroke Primer – my version

Disclaimer: Please understand that my presentation of the following stroke information is a description of my own interpretation based on what I have read and experienced. I am in a non-medical profession and had a stroke nearly 5 years ago. What I've learned on this 4.5-year journey is more information about strokes than I ever would have wanted. For technical and scientific information, I urge you to find online sources. Most of the numbers I refer to in this chapter are from a 2011 publication of the National Stroke Association (NSA); I tried to find more recent data, but all I located was a 2014 publication with 2010 data. My advice is to do your own research and find your own answers because most of the information I found did not come from my health-care providers. What medical professionals know about stroke can be summarized by an often-repeated statement: "Every patient is different, every stroke is different, and every recovery is different." I find this answer dissatisfying.

What I've discovered since the stroke is that there's a need for more research into preventing brain injury (and resulting disability) during and just after stroke. There is a drug (tPA) that can be used within the first few hours of an ischemic stroke, but it was not given to me. There's nothing that can be done now for the damage to my brain, but a new treatment could prevent disability in future stroke patients. Another area that's lacking solutions is in recovery from hemiparesis, a common disability caused by stroke. These are where attention (money) is needed: either how to prevent the disability or how to rehab from the disability.

As for me, my focus has always been on rehabilitation, not research into stroke prevention or disability prevention.

I want to be successful recovering my lost abilities – no more, no less. But no effective therapy exists.

If you have survived a stroke and have hemiparesis, please understand that just because there is no known treatment that is effective for most survivors, doesn't mean you won't recover. What it means that no one is going to give you a protocol to follow that is likely to result in 100% recovery. What you will need to do is to cobble together exercises and treatments that you can – and will – do on your own, then do them.

This is my simplistic explanation of stroke:

There are two types of strokes, with two different causes, but both resulting in the same condition because they both deprive an area - or multiple areas - of the brain of the oxygen necessary for survival of the brain cells. The two types are (1) ischemic, caused by a blockage in a blood vessel that prevents oxygen from making it to its assigned cells, and (2) hemorrhagic (a.k.a., bleeding), caused by the rupture of the wall of a blood vessel in the brain, which floods an area of the brain, preventing oxygen absorption. Both circumstances result in dead and/or damaged brain cells.

The blockage in the former (#1 above) can be caused by a blood clot or a piece of plaque (formed on the walls of arteries).

A bleeding stroke (#2 above) is caused by a rupture, of a blood vessel, a brain hemorrhage. Ruptures occur at weak spots in a blood vessel, including at arteriovenous malformations (AVM), a congenital condition that constitutes just a handful of the total number of strokes.

The resulting oxygen deprivation in both stroke types causes two kinds of damage: the killing of one or more areas of the brain and the stunning of nearby areas (called the penumbra). The dead cells will never be revived, while the penumbra cells often do recover, sometimes spontaneously, without any therapy and sometimes with therapy.

To recover the functions formerly controlled by the dead areas, a formerly unused area of the brain must be recruited to do so; the areas in the penumbra might recover. Both types of damage can be compensated for by dint of repetition – or attempted repetition – of a function.

The numbers

Stroke is the fourth leading cause of death in the United States. Just under 800,000 Americans have strokes each year, that is, 1 every 40 seconds. To date, stroke survivors in the United States total 7 million.

Why more research has not been done into preventing damage immediately following a stroke or into more effective rehabilitation is beyond my understanding: the health cost burden for stroke survivors adds up to at least $32 billion per year, including $73.7 billion in 2010. Given that most business decisions are based on economics, I would think at least insurance companies and/or the federal government (because of Medicare) would invest more into research to save themselves billions of dollars every month. But that's not the case. Money is invested in stroke awareness and preventing stroke, but not enough goes into preventing immediate damage (the cascade of death of neurons) or into rehab, which is why the mantra

"Every stroke is different ..." is often repeated. Yes, the statement is true, but it's also content-free. It roughly translates into, "I don't know," and every single member of your health-care team (current and future) will say that to you.

The Smoking Gun

When a patient has been identified as having had a stroke, one of the first things medical personnel do is look for the smoking gun, evidence of what has caused the stroke, physically how the stroke happened. One of the first things a patient does is ask, "Why/How did this happen?"

Of course, the survivor's question has two meanings: (1) the physical/mechanical - "How did this happen?" (the equivalent of the neurologist's smoking gun) and (2) the metaphysical - "Why did this happen to *me*?" Clearly the answer to the latter is as unanswerable as, "Who am I?" and "Why am I here?" Religion, accepting that the trauma has a purpose, helps some people find answers, as does focusing on gratitude and recognizing blessings.

Finding the smoking gun is what many doctors excel at: solving a puzzle by piecing together bits of information that coalesce into a logical, albeit esoteric, explanation. Plus, it begs the patient's second question, which often blames the victim, or is outside the scope of a physician's training.

The book "Blaming the Victim" was written by William Ryan in 1971. The book's premise has stayed with me since I read it for a sociology class in college. Throughout the 30 years following, I have found probably a hundred confirmations of his theory.

Ryan's thesis is that people who end up in bad circumstances – economically or as the target of crime (in the wrong neighborhood, alone in the dark, for example) – are ultimately responsible for the bad results themselves.

Let's forget the economic part (which is Ryan's focus), and take up how it applies to health:

An obese person is blamed for any medical problem that develops. People who have high cholesterol and high blood pressure were just setting themselves up for having a stroke. Alcoholics bring on their own cirrhosis; smokers, their lung cancer.

Personally, as much as I fight it, I fall into thinking the same way. It happens every time I think along the lines of: I was super-fit, at my perfect weight, and had low cholesterol and blood pressure at the time I had the stroke, but I caused it myself by straining while rowing. In fact, it even seems ironic because, given my age, my health and my lifestyle, I did not "deserve" the stroke. Those overweight people who eat french fries and also smoke – they're the ones who should be having strokes.

Another easy way of blaming the victim comes about when the stroke survivor had a genetic defect that caused a bleeding stroke.

Blaming the victim is a way people have of denying their own risk, of maintaining the comforting delusion that they are in control of their futures, that heart disease, stroke, cancer and other nasties will not get them as long as they stay slim, eat a healthy diet (low in fat, high in fiber, with 8 glasses of water daily) and get enough cardiovascular exercise.

From the ER at our local hospital, I was sent for a CT scan right away. Thank God my husband walked into the ER saying, "My wife had a stroke, my wife had a stroke," so that I didn't spend time waiting or undergoing tests wondering what the diagnosis was. Everyone there was shocked to see me wheeled in as the "wife who was having a stroke." Even with my gray hair, I was far too young for that. Now I know that *in utero* babies sometimes have strokes – and toddlers, school-aged children, teenagers and college students. Not just elderly women or overweight smokers.

My CT scan showed that my right carotid artery was blocked, so we had that piece of the puzzle right away. Another CT scan and an MRI showed why - that my right carotid artery had been "dissected," that is, the internal lining had separated from the wall and fallen across the interior, blocking blood flow. Dissections often occur as the result of physical strain – for example, trying to lift something too hard for the person to lift (weightlifters and rowers are prime examples).

For other patients, the search for the smoking gun might lead to locating the source of a bleed – where the vessel burst - and whether repair is needed to stop the bleeding.

A friend from high school had a stroke around the same time that I did; she had an ischemic stroke caused by a blood clot thrown off by a malignant tumor on one of her ovaries. Her attitude was that having a stroke had a significant upside – it saved her from dying of ovarian cancer. My reaction was sympathy for her having to undergo chemotherapy during her first year of stroke recovery. Even without chemo, my first year was hell.

In the ER, after finding the clot in my carotid artery, one of the docs told me that the only treatment they had was giving me tPA (tissue plasmogen activator), but it was too "dangerous," and then did not explain the danger. I had a vague memory of hearing of a treatment that had to be given within a few hours of the stroke, but not the details.

So, let me get this straight: a woman comes to the ER *having* a stroke, with stroke symptoms coming and going, and they ask her to approve not treating her because it was too dangerous to receive long after the onset of the stroke? My husband and I both went for what the expert advised.

We later found out that tPA is a clot-busting drug and perhaps might have helped, but there's no way of knowing. Except that, according to my husband, the "no tPA" decision was made during one of my periods of being able to squeeze fingers, when the doctor was saying it might not have been a stroke after all, but rather some transient ischemic event (TIA) that would result in little to no damage. Wrong. In that case, tPA would have been unnecessary and dangerous, as determined.

Also, although I look at myself as being in the process of having a stroke when I appeared at the ER (because my symptoms were intermittent, as though the damage was happening right then), there are indications that the stroke happened promptly after the Plymouth race, and that we ignored the early symptoms – stumbling; slurred speech; swelling around my right eye, which one neurologist later told me could have been due to blood backed up into the artery surrounding my eye, backed up from the block in my carotid artery. Those symptoms started appearing 5 days before I showed up in the ER, too long before to allow the use of tPA, which must be administered within 3 hours after the onset of the stroke.

It turns out that our local hospital was recently given a superb grade for the survival rate of stroke patients. I was not treated in its ER, but was shipped to Massachusetts General the following morning. I survived, but with a significant disability. My opinion is that, given the increasing occurrence of stroke, much more research must be done regarding preventing the damage that is taking place between the onset of the stroke and settling into the post-acute stage – that is, preventing what's called the "cascade of death" that finishes off some of the cells in the penumbra. I am convinced that the brain damage I had happened while I was under medical supervision. My situation might have been entirely different if there had been something that could have been done for me between the time I showed up in the ER and the permanent damage that was done.

I don't mean to imply that anything was done wrong in the ER. I received the best treatment possible based on the standard of care at the time. Unfortunately, nothing has changed in the years since then, and someone having a comparable stroke today would receive exactly the same care, with the same disability as a result.

One problem with trying to unambiguously identify the smoking gun in my case was the lapse in time between the artery dissection (whenever that was) and having the permanent brain damage. I think the row in which I broke the pin was the hardest I strained during the period preceding the stroke, but that was about two weeks before my symptoms. The come-from-behind row was the final one before the stroke; but even that was 5 days before conventional symptoms appeared.

Bottom line: it may be that I was showing stroke symptoms without anyone recognizing them as such until that morning 5 days after the dissection when I presented conventional symptoms.

Unlike in my situation, in some stroke cases, no explanation is ever found – no broken blood vessel or clot. Disturbingly, the "Why/How did this happen?" question is just never answered. As much as I've resented the "every stroke is different," answer, not knowing the mechanics of the stroke I had would have driven me beyond crazy. Even with all I *do* know about the stroke I had, I still resent not knowing which rowing incident broke my artery. It will always be a guess, which irritates me.

So far, three things about the current medical situation concerning stroke frustrate me: (1) there was no way of successfully treating me in the ER; (2) there was no way of stopping the death of the large part of my brain that died in the hours just after the stroke; and (3) there is no post-stroke rehab therapy that is likely to work *and* there's little-to-no research into rehab.

Numbers 1 and 2 mean that more brain damage was caused than had to be, resulting in more severe disability. Number 3 means that I'm on my own as far as recovery goes, that my success in rehab -just like every other survivor's success - is a do-it-yourself situation.

I know that all patients have to advocate for themselves when it comes to treatment for any medical issue, but stroke rehab is ridiculously lacking: here we are, with absolutely no therapy that is likely to work, brain-damaged with no knowledge about treatments, and a lack of information from medical personnel. Realistically, there are lots of therapies to try out, but you are best off finding what combination works for you. As for myself, in my quest for recovery, desperation took me on many tangential paths. I have tried nearly every healing method I've heard about.

I recently wrote in my blog about this DIY situation ...

DIY Medical Treatment

Posted June 2014

... As much as I hope and pray for a miracle stroke recovery protocol, the best I can do now is incorporate my new condition into my life as it is.

I don't mean to encourage losing hope, but ... I'm hedging my bets. I'm living my little life being as happy and productive as I can. I don't expect a magic pill or invention that will bring on my full recovery, but I will plod along doing the available therapies as hard as I can, always hoping for the best return. And if a "cure" comes along, all the better...

Managing stroke disabilities means developing a way of life that works for the survivor ...

Stroke survivors investigate available therapies and see what works for them. Sound do-it-yourself? It is.

We use our doctors and medical personnel as advisors and resources, but ultimately make the decisions ourselves, based on the, albeit incomplete, information we gather.

Back to my experience in the ER:

In summary, in the Addison-Gilbert ER, my CT scan resulted in the ER doctor telling me that I'd had an ischemic stroke caused by the dissection of my right carotid artery. The one-cell-thick lining ("think Saran Wrap," he said) of my artery had ruptured away from the artery wall and collapsed across the vessel. Blood continued up the artery until it was blocked, and it clotted there. (Although my husband disputes it), the doctor said that the top edge of the clot had a ragged upper end and, with my blood as "sticky" as it was, the blood that was making it past the clot was snagging bits off the ragged end and "spewing" them into the right side of my brain. Not an encouraging bit of information.

While in the ER, I was tested repeatedly: "Who's the president of the United States?" "What's today's date?" "Can you move your toes?" and, after the doctor carefully put his first two fingers in my left hand, "Can you squeeze my fingers?"

The squeezing test was repeated frequently because sometimes I could do it, but sometimes I could not. When I couldn't, as when I first arrived, the doctor and my husband would look very worried; when I could, their relief was evident.

Until the CT scan, they were calling my condition a series of TIAs (transient ischemic attacks, a.k.a. mini-strokes, which leave little or no lasting damage). Now, admit it, doesn't a "mini-stroke" sound much less threatening than a "stroke"?

In fact, by the time Tom called my boss to say I would not be at the office that day, he called what was happening a "mini-stroke," which somehow morphed into a "minor stroke" by the time my boss told my co-workers why I was out. Called a "minor" stroke, I don't think any of my co-workers expected the magnitude of my resulting disability.

From that point on, after seeing how incapacitated I was by the event, Tom started calling it a "severe" stroke, which I hated, since I'd simply had a stroke and my brain was injured, the extent of which was no one's business except mine and my family's. As it turns out, a truly "severe" stroke kills far more brain cells and results in coma and/or death, or living with far more limitations than I have – the inability to walk, sometimes even to swallow or eat. The extent of the stroke I had was along the lines of, as someone said (but I don't remember who), having "lost a lot of real estate." Survivors themselves often refer to the "massive stroke" they had. The one I had was absolutely *not* massive. What is this, a competition?

The stroke I had whacked the entire right side of my brain, but given the resulting damage, I haven't ever called it "severe" or "massive." The resulting damage: left hemiparesis (weakness on my left side, because it is controlled by the right side of my brain, where the damage was). This included the total inability to use my left side, other than using my hip flexor to dominate enough synergistic movement to swing my leg brace (an "ankle-foot orthotic," aka, AFO)-encased leg forward in order to take a step. I was never near death, never couldn't be myself there inside my unresponsive body, never couldn't hear, speak or eat. Physically, I could do everything except use my left side. Not too bad, I'd say, especially since I'm right-handed. Mentally, I had lost significant executive functioning, but after a couple of days, I could still factor a quadratic equation (although, again, my husband disputes my memory). That loss of executive functions resulted in my inability to adequately perform my job, but I *couldn't tell*, because of a particular part of my brain having been damaged.

The following June (7 months post-stroke), I wrote this blog entry about the problem.

Anosognosia [or Agnosia]

Posted 22nd June 2010

When my cognitive abilities were evaluated after the stroke, one of my identified problems was called Anosognosia [a.k.a. agnosia], a condition my neurologist defined as "generally used to signify not understanding the extent or significance of one's deficits." In other words, I suffer from the inability to recognize my limitations caused by the stroke. In some brain-injured people, this phenomenon results in some significant risk-taking behaviors - like continuing to drive after having a stroke.

My reality was that even the morning I had the stroke, I didn't recognize any drastic change from what was normal inside my head. Sure, I had trouble putting weight on my left ankle so that I fell over whenever I stood on my own ... plus I had a mild headache right behind my right eye (when I never had headaches [before]). But those were all physical issues; everything inside my brain - thinking, feeling and logic - felt normal and has continued to do so. That's a symptom, I suspect, of the anosognosia condition - I don't feel incapable of thinking clearly and figuring out things as I used to - I have retained my ingrained "How hard can it be?" attitude. I observe that I make more mistakes now and for a while, calendars were far more baffling than they used to be. Maps and spatial relationships, as always, continue to confound me. Recovering cognitively is much harder for me to assess compared to recovering physically - if I can lift the yellow ball with both arms, I can see that today I am capable of more than I was in December, but, if all along I have been clueless about the whack my cognitive skills took, how do I assess progress? I am pleased that I can usually complete the daily crossword puzzle in the Gloucester Daily Times and I can often complete the Cry[p]toquote, but ... I was not able to come anywhere near completing the crossword puzzle in the Sunday Boston Globe, something that I did regularly before the stroke - it might have taken me the whole week, but I generally completed it every week.

For me, another effect of having anosognosia was my inability to accept that my sense of touch was gone on my left side. Every time anyone tested me for feeling in my affected side, I went along, my brain thinking I could feel their touch on my arm or leg. When my proprioception (the ability to tell where a part of my body was located in space) was tested, I came up with answers I believed.

For example, with my arm on a table in front of me (where I could see it), I was supposed to tell the tester whether I could feel a touch. You know what? I was convinced I could and said "yes" each time I was touched. Then the tester told me to close my eyes so that we could do it again; each time I felt something, I said, "yes." No one ever told me when I performed correctly, but I truly thought I did okay, even though sometimes I didn't feel much (as though I was a bit numb) and thought I might be guessing.

There was also a test in which my hand was on the table, my eyes were closed, and each of my fingers was raised and lowered and I was to say "up" or "down" based on what I felt; sometimes I really couldn't tell, but answered anyway.

Every time someone touched me on my leg and he/she asked if I could feel it, I *could*, and I said so. And I was convinced I could until a neurologist came into my room and repeatedly poked my leg with a pin. Even though I watched him do it, I didn't even flinch, which at the time, I realized was the wrong reaction. Agnosia.

One aspect of anosognosia is knowing the information, but being in denial about it; maybe I was in denial rather than being dishonest.

I kept asking my physiatrist (the doc who manages your rehab while you're in the hospital and after) why I seemed so much worse off than the other patients at Spaulding (not including those still fighting for their lives in Intensive Care at MGH), why my roommate could hold onto a walker with both hands. Why did some survivors need an AFO to walk, but could use the hand on that side, etc.? In addition to the standard "every stroke is different …every recovery is different" answer, he finally beckoned me and my husband to follow him. We ended up at a computer on which he retrieved an MRI of my brain taken on Day 1. He called the whitish shadowy area the "affected" part of my brain – it went fully front to back and side to side inside my skull; the left side of my brain had no white/gray. There was the answer literally in black and white. - no wonder I was having such a hard time.

Immediately Post-Stroke

When I was first disabled, I could not be left alone unless lying in bed. Even lying in bed, the nurses didn't trust me and left on a bed alarm that was activated if I sat on the edge of the bed. I was labeled "impulsive" because I wanted to do what I wanted to do, and, if I could, I would – or at least attempt to – do it. To the Spaulding staff, I was not safe alone anywhere. Nurses had to be with me no matter what, unless I was lying in bed. Bathroom, time sitting in a chair - a nurse and/or therapist had to help me not fall while I moved around. Their preferred location for me was either in my bed or off in the gym doing therapy with a therapist.

To shower, I had to find a nurse willing to roll my wheelchair into the shower room, stay there and help scrub me, getting her rubber-soled shoes wet.

After a couple of days, they trained my husband to help transfer me from bed to wheelchair and wheelchair to toilet, and even gave him permission to roll me down the hall to the alternate restroom, which had a toilet that was a better height for me. He was not allowed to help me shower, though – that was far too dangerous.

Once Tom passed muster by demonstrating he could safely (for both me and his back) transfer me, the information on my white board was changed to say so.

Each patient's white board listed what the patient was capable of. Basically, it said I needed help with everything (bathroom, dressing, shower, etc.), and I could eat whatever I wanted. Whenever I asked a nurse or aide for something, his/her eyes would flick up to the white board to check if it was okay. I was interested in the patient across the hall.

From my bed, I could see a huge "I" on her white board, and asked someone what it meant. "Independent" was the answer – the patient was allowed to do whatever she wanted all by herself, no monitor needed. I was envious until I realized her situation. She was a 20-year-old college student who was competent enough to leave, but the hospital wouldn't release her until her college came up with a handicapped-accessible dorm room appropriate for her abilities. That was one of many times I've thought, "It could be worse." It happened again when it was time for my roommate to be discharged. She had been able to walk by herself and go to the bathroom by herself already when I moved into the room 4 weeks previously). She had family – some grown kids, their spouses and her grandkids – who came to visit one evening a week. But when she was ready to leave, there was nowhere for her to live. Her social worker would visit every day and run through a list of the nursing homes she had called but no one had room for her. I was humiliated for her. Again, I was reminded that my situation could have been worse. I had a husband who wanted to take me home and was willing to be my caregiver; and I had siblings willing to care for me when I first went home, freeing Tom to go back to working full-time.

I want to be brutally honest in this account of my recovery, despite any reader's squeamishness. Going to the bathroom with someone else in the room was humiliating; urinating is fine, but having a bowel movement is awful, especially because one of my meds was a stool softener that made my stool gooey and barely controllable. Nurses would help me remove my sometimes-soiled panties, and often could not restrain their disgust. At least I could wipe myself.

I have always had a long-term plan for my career, which included productive and rewarding work as a writer, including writing a novel that ends up on *The New York Times* bestseller list. Managing a newspaper, which was my job at the time of the stroke, was not part of that plan. My short-term plans all related to inching along toward what I wanted in the long-term.

Post-stroke, that long-term writing goal remains the same.

But my short-term goals changed as soon as I had the stroke. In addition to marching along toward my long-term goals, I now have many shorter-term physical goals imposed by the stroke, including being able to (1) participate in my favorite sports (primarily rowing) and other activities (hiking, gardening, serious cooking and baking, along with working on home improvements), as I used to, and (2) safely walk anywhere without a cane so that I can carry things or walk my dog; and tasks that require the use of both hands. These are activities that were automatic for me pre-stroke, but daunting post-stroke.

Please note that "automatic," means "taken for granted."

And, just as they were pre-stroke, both my long-term and short-term goals are possible, but not guaranteed. Remember that there are no guarantees – not in my post-stroke future and/or recovery, just as there were none in my pre-stroke future.

Intermission I: I was just thinking ... about disabilities

(originally published in the Community Advocate newspaper, 2012)

Everyone has challenges and they span a wide spectrum: medical, physical, psychological, circumstance. And everyone responds differently – from resigned acceptance to fighting mad. I have a physical challenge: I am disabled – half-paralyzed by a stroke two-and-a-half years ago. I have struggled to recover as much function as I can, while the medical community says that I have finished improving, that no stroke survivor does after two years post-stroke. Although others might define my situation differently, I find that my challenge is working hard toward an unknown endpoint.

People often believe that "everything happens for a reason." By that, they are not referring to the physiology or mechanics of what happened, but rather, the underlying philosophical reason, which makes me look for beneficial results of my disability, positive things that have come out of this nightmare: gratitude, how to be encouraging, appreciation for minuscule improvements, acknowledgement that before the stroke I had the best life ever.

I have a friend who was brain injured during a carjacking. Although I did not know her before her injury, she is convinced that the reason it happened to her was because she was irritable, impatient, and misguided enough to fight the carjackers, which is what led to her broken skull. Now she is a sweet, mild-mannered woman I call when I need encouragement. She believes her transformation came about because she needed to learn that material possessions have no importance and that her role is to be kind and to care about others. She learned it.

After the injury, B was told that she would never walk unaided again. You know what? She walks many miles every day without any brace or cane and doesn't even limp. When I met her, I couldn't tell she'd been brain-injured; I just knew that she could not work or drive, but not the reason.

After the stroke I had, a neurologist told my husband that, at best, I would only ever use my paralyzed leg as a peg, and going up and down stairs would be out of the question so I would have to sleep on the first floor of our house. You know what? My gait is terrible and I cannot lift my knee straight up as though I'm marching, but I can bend my knee [slightly] and I can climb any stairs I encounter – both feet on each step - as long as I have my cane; in fact, I once went up more than 100 steps at an old castle in Sweden; I eventually stopped counting because I had proved my point (to myself).

I often think that the best thing a disabled person can hear is that he/she will never walk again. I have observed that as the best motivator of all; it brings out the "fighting mad" reaction.

A friend told me the story of a man who had a stroke and was told he'd never walk again; six months later, he walked his daughter down the aisle at her wedding.

A disability is like a gauntlet, a dare to accomplish what people tell us is impossible, a challenge to bring out the best in each of us, an opportunity to experience gratitude.

And those who are not disabled can work on being grateful too.

Recovery

Recovery therapy

A stroke survivor's therapy invariably starts in rehab. While in rehab immediately post-stroke, I had a schedule set that included an hour each day of: physical, occupational, speech and language, and recreational therapy.

Physical therapy (PT) includes your body below the waist, primarily your legs, with the focus on walking. Occupational (OT) works on above your waist (i.e., your arm and hand) and includes relearning how to perform activities of daily living (ADL's), like dressing. Speech and language (SL) helps with exactly what it's called – while a right-side stroke slaps the daylights out of some cognitive skills, a left-side stroke affects your language center, sometimes resulting in aphasia, difficulty speaking. Also, the first thing my SL therapist did was sit next to me with some crackers and a cup of water for a swallowing assessment; I started by sipping the water – no problem; she then handed me a graham cracker, followed by a Saltine – I chewed small pieces of them carefully, mixing in lots of saliva to keep from inhaling a crumb, and I had no trouble with those either. That meant I'd be able to be on an unrestricted diet, selecting whatever I wanted to eat from a regular menu.

I was allowed everything, including dessert every dinner – in fact, I think I could have had it for lunch *and* dinner. And my PT was concerned about my unused muscles atrophying, so I was encouraged to maintain my weight. Eating dessert made that easier, although it did nothing to prevent muscle loss, just resulted in an increase of fat.

By the time I was released from the rehab hospital, I had lost 10 pounds, but all muscle. I think I had just as much fat on my body as when I went in, or maybe more. I know I lost significant muscle through atrophy from non-use: I had no gluteus muscles on my left side (even now, sitting on a hard surface is brutal) and my left forearm is a skin-covered bone that reminds me of a chicken wing.

Obviously, every pound of fat/weight gained is one that must be shed as a survivor recovers, but being disabled interferes with the best way to lose weight – doing an exercise you love. Being fit pre-stroke was easy compared to post-stroke: my favorites - running and rowing - became out of the question for me. Even four-and-a-half years post-stroke, the limit of what I can do: walk, row on a rowing machine, ride a stationary bike, and water-walk, but none of my former exercising. I would probably be able to use an elliptical trainer if only I weren't so afraid of it.

My unsolicited advice, then, is to find an exercise (even a compromise, like a rowing machine instead of rowing) you enjoy – and (per Nike) "Just Do It." It will be good for your health *and* your recovery.

If you never exercised or played a sport pre-stroke, you are unlikely to do so post-stroke, per stroke guru Peter Levine. Do what you can do safely, though. And enjoy it so that you continue doing it.

One more bit of advice: If anyone *ever* says the word "plateau" to you, jettison him/her as an advisor. The concept behind the word is that a survivor has improved as much as possible in a particular area and, no matter what, cannot improve farther. That is, bluntly, bullshit. Progress stops when *you* stop, when you give up. And, as we all know, we must "never give up."

The bottom line is that you are the one with the most invested in your recovery, the most to lose by not recovering, so you must be your own advocate for continuing on and expecting to make progress. You may have medical professionals telling you that your progress is over, that every ability you will ever get back happens in the first six months, year, or two years. If they do, they are wrong. Perhaps they are saying it because your insurance visits are running out. Believing those plateau-pushers will only discourage you, make you doubt your optimism, and wonder why you're wasting so much time on recovery exercises, when it is not actually time wasted, but time (and repetitions) invested.

What hitting a plateau really means is that your current therapy approach has helped you as much as it can, and to keep improving, you must change your approach.

As for different types of therapy, after getting the advice of your medical team, you are best off investigating methods yourself and using the ones that are appealing – and possible – for you. These could be the ones with the most scientific support for effectiveness, or the cheapest, or the ones that fit into your routine and you are most likely to do. Remember that it's your choice.

There are dozens of approaches you can try, and if your therapists don't know about all of them, you can find out about them by doing a little research yourself – talk to other therapists you encounter, chat on online stroke forums, with other survivors, and *read*. Be sure to read everything you can about stroke - books and/or blogs about brain research or stroke, by experts and by survivors. No matter how educated a stroke expert is, only stroke survivors are true experts on the topic of recovery. There are lots of us online, and we are generally opinionated about the experiences and medical treatment we've had.

In addition to conventional exercises, you might want to look into electronic stimulation (eStim), mirror therapy, Botox, constraint-induced (or modified constraint-induced) therapy, and aquatic therapy, along with various limb-specific hardware, like Saebo and Bioness products. There are survivors who swear by yoga, acupuncture and/or chiropractic treatment. Some of these therapies are not covered by insurance plans, but you might be in the financial position to pay for them yourself.

Insurance is one of the factors in determining how long (in calendar time) and what avenues you can use as you pursue recovery. Some insurance policies cover a certain total number of therapy sessions, while others will cover therapy only in the first two years, etc. All require that "progress" as objectively evaluated by your therapist, be made.

Your therapists will help you set goals (e.g., donning and removing your shoes, particularly tricky if you wear an ankle-foot orthotic (AFO); successfully doing that shows progress. If it takes 100 practice attempts before you successfully get your shoes on, do it 100 times, and more. What you need is to be able to get on your shoes by yourself when you want to. That's what you want, and what your insurance company wants.

To receive as much therapy as possible paid for by your insurance company, make sure you understand what your insurance covers and how to ensure that each session is covered (Do you need a referral or some approval beforehand? Is the therapy method approved for coverage given your condition?) Understand that some insurance companies routinely deny re-imbursement for perfectly acceptable treatment; the company is betting that some of their clients will accept the company's first decision, give up, and not contest the decision. Always contest a denial so that your therapy session gets a second look. Sometimes the denial is for a valid reason, but sometimes it's an arbitrary decision, a knee-jerk "no," to test your resolve.

Recovering Activities of Daily Living

Dressing

Ranking the returning responsibilities for being capable of the "activities of daily living" (ADL's), being allowed to go to the bathroom by myself was at the top of the list for me. Dressing myself was the next.

Obviously men and women have different challenges in this ADL, although there is some overlap, like tying sneakers and putting on shirts. On the plus side for both genders: all of us have the help of lower expectations from others *and* from ourselves. For a long time, we don't even have to *try* to get dressed up for fancy occasions. Actually, we get to even wear the same clothes for days in a row, plus sleep in our clothes. Confession time: Early on, putting on bras was such a struggle for me that once I had one on, it was on for at least two days – through the nights, too. Now I go without, unless a bra is absolutely necessary (in my view) under the top.

Every stroke survivor learns how to dress in rehab. We don't necessarily get enough practice there because it's much easier for the aide who is helping us get up and ready to do a lot of it herself. (Remember: isn't it easier to dress a two-year-old yourself?) Not only is the aide under the gun to have us ready by the time our first therapist appears at the door to wheel us to the gym, she also must have other patients ready-to-go at their appropriate times. That meant that, although I passed each dressing test individually (pulling a shirt on over my head, getting my panties on, pulling on sweatpants and then the shoes and socks routine), getting the whole process completed by myself was a different story. My last day in rehab, the aide abandoned me mid-sponge bath and never returned; that was the first time in over a month that I had to get dressed entirely by myself. I wondered if it was on purpose in order to see if I could, and it took me forever, but I managed without anyone's help. Finishing the sponge bath was the hardest because it was cold and the rinse water was out of my reach. By the end of dressing I was very frustrated and was starting to doubt myself: I had fought very hard for my health team to finally agree to release me, but maybe they were right to be dragging their feet. If I couldn't even dress myself without enormous frustration, why was I going home anyway?

There are just a couple of keys to getting dressed; once a survivor knows those, some frustrations are alleviated.

The affected limb goes first into a garment. It doesn't matter if you just spent 50 years with the routine of putting your right leg first into your pants, you will now put it in first only if it's your affected one. Same for shirts, sweaters, jackets. The one exception to this rule is that the first sock and shoe go on your unaffected leg – so that you have a firm support pushing against the floor while you put your shoe and sock on the affected side.

Also, I have found it warmer to dress my bottom half first, including shoes, then don my top.

When you put your affected arm into a top, you must get the sleeve on at least up to your elbow before trying to get your unaffected arm in. BTW, the inside entry hole of sleeves on your unaffected side is always much higher and more behind you than you think, so twist your shoulder farther back or reach up behind your head as you poke your hand around trying to find the sleeve.

Use your teeth when it would help. My first outpatient OT told me, "Forget what your grandma told you about your teeth – 'They're jewels, not tools.' You *will* be using your teeth as tools." Teeth are especially handy for pulling the sleeve of a long-sleeved shirt off your unaffected arm when you undress.

Don't expect your pre-stroke favorites in your wardrobe to even be acceptable post-stroke; each item will have its own idiosyncrasies that can make it unwearable. The single most important characteristic I found that determined whether I could wear a pre-stroke favorite was the fabric's stretchiness. Cotton dresses were the first to be axed unless the neckline and waist were wide enough for me to step into and pull up, which is true only of those few that button all the way up the front. Buttons also determine whether I can put it on by myself. I have found zippers to be impossible when I have to put the ends together to get it started; large buttons are better than small; slightly looser buttonholes are easier than those just larger than the button. If you have someone else helping you dress, by all means, wear whatever they can help you get into.

I suggest starting each day by dressing yourself, but not getting trapped in your shirt. Dressing myself made me start the day feeling empowered, despite the fact I was so pathetically dependent in so many other ways. Be proud of yourself if you can get up in the morning, pick out appropriate clothes for your activities that day, and then dress yourself without crying (or swearing). That is a huge accomplishment! Brag if you are a woman and can don a bathing suit (a dry one-piece one).

If pre-stroke you showered every morning, you might want to change your standards; dressing while you're damp is the worst, even if you use baby powder. Without taking a shower, you can correct your bed-head by sticking your head under a faucet. Women: keep your hair short if you like how it looks that way and, if it's gray, dye it if that

55

makes you feel better about your appearance. Ditto re make-up: Apply whatever makes you feel better about yourself, but be careful not to poke yourself in the eye with the mascara wand or eyeliner. You have enough medical problems and don't need to create more.

I had certain dressing milestones along the way, one described in this entry from 4 months post-stroke:

clothes

13th February 2010

For the first time in three months, I'm wearing jeans! It's an experiment to see whether I can manage them when I go to the bathroom - that's the litmus test these days. For the past three months, my pants have been limited to sweats, flannel pajama pants and other pants that have elastic or drawstrings at the waist so that I can pull them both down and up one-handed when I go to the bathroom. At first, I had just one pair [of] flowered sweat pants that Millie had approved about six months ago when we were shopping together –

Back then, "If you wear those," she said, nodding at a rack in the store, "you'll be the coolest mother ever," so I found the right size and bought them. I couldn't wear them at the rehab hospital, though, because my PT objected to how thick the fabric was when she clamped on the Locomat assistive walking device. So Tom and my sister Beth went shopping for me and ended up with two pairs of navy blue jersey tie-string exercise pants. In the rehab hospital, Tom brought in clothes every day for me to wear the following day, left neatly folded in a stack in my closet. As long as the items were in a pile, the nurses could pull out the stack when it was time for me to get dressed; at that point, the nurse would hold up each item and ask if I wanted to wear it today. Whatever it was, I nodded or said yes because that was what Tom had brought in. On the days he made a mistake and brought only one sock, the nurse of the day would grumble, but I would tell them I could wear socks from yesterday. [Yes, it was in the rehab hospital that my cleanliness standards started to slip] Eventually, Tom brought in extra socks so that there were alternatives in case of a mistake. Each day, Tom diligently took home my clothes from the previous day ...and brought in a clean set for the following day. And he brought in my favorite red flannel nightshirt so that I had cuddly pj's to sleep in. Tom has been diligent throughout this ordeal, but the most diligent was in those days when he would gather up my clothes from the laundry room at home, pack up and head for work at 8 a.m., then leave work at 3:30 p.m. to go to the hospital to see me, sit through my various therapies, help me with dinner and catching up on e-mail, then hang out with me until about 7:30, when he would head home, start a load of laundry, if needed, then get up in the morning to start over again, day after day of having little choice in how he was going to spend his [time]. It was that steadfast diligence that has helped me keep upbeat throughout this ordeal - and he wonders sometimes how I can remain so sunny and optimistic - when the reality is that I do it for him - I do it because it makes it all worth it for him. The trick is just focusing on all the wonderful things in my life - him, our kids, friends, the beautiful earth, exercise, sunshine, my job, chocolate, flowers, dogs, good books, music and progress ...

Back to the jeans: Last week, I met a woman at OT who was wearing jean capris. When she explained to the OT why she was there, it was to get her left arm back to doing the things it could do before the stroke. When we talked to each other, she said that her stroke had occurred in December - a month after [I had one]

57

- and there she was, still one-handed - wearing non-elastic-waistband pants. That's when my jeans daydreams started. Going along with it is the idea that I will one day be able to pick out my own clothes in the morning. Don't get me wrong - it's not that I wear things I don't want to wear - Tom is very good about asking for my input, but it's a lot like letting a 2-year-old pick out her own clothes - this shirt or that one? And the pants choice is always between the navy exercise or the plaid flannel - on special occasions, it's the black sweats. As soon as I mentioned the woman in jeans to him, Tom has been planning for the day he would offer me the choice of jeans. To fit over my brace, they are his jeans, not my own - and he mentioned last week that it would be today, if I were up for it.

As I said, the litmus test is whether I can button and zip them myself, so after getting them on this morning, we tried that and it worked fine the first try. Once I was downstairs, though, I went to the bathroom and could NOT get the button done one-handed. I called Tom to the bathroom, where he straightened out the waistband (which was bunched up) and buttoned and zippered them. Horrifyingly, I started to cry because, as I said, "How come I could do it upstairs, but not downstairs? I thought this was progress - I don't want to be going backwards. I've gone backwards far enough."

He hugged me and gave me a pep talk - of course I wasn't going backwards, of course if I could do it upstairs, I could - and would - do it again wherever I was. He then explained that the difference was that I hadn't made sure the waistband was smooth before trying to close the front.

It's important to remember that once you have accomplished something, if you persist, you will continue to be able to do it in the future. There is a danger, though, of thinking that if you do something once, it's a permanent part of your repertoire; it's not, unless you continue doing it, unless you get enough practice to do it reliably. In the case of my jeans, there was still a lot of progress to be made: wearing my own loosest jeans, not Tom's; struggling by myself to button and zip, if that's what it took; and wearing jeans frequently. Also, it helped if I wore the same pair of jeans more than one day: given the way jeans stretch, they are looser Day 2, then even more on Day 3, etc. Along the same line, don't put your jeans in the dryer after you wash them – use a cold-water wash and then line dry them so that they don't shrink. They will be crisp and wrinkled, but you'll be able to close them by yourself.

If you have an AFO with a bottom bigger than the sole of your foot, most of your favorite old shoes will be out of the question. You might have sneakers that stretch enough to accommodate your new gigantic foot apparatus; I didn't. For the first several months post-stroke, I wore an old sneaker on my unaffected right foot and one of Tom's on my left foot and AFO; then we settled for buying two pairs of the same type of shoe – a 7 for my right foot and a 9 for my left. It was such a waste [of money and resources], and looked ridiculous, that I bought double shoes only twice. It took me a long time (1.5 years) to devise a solution so that I could wear shoes that didn't look ridiculous. My solution was when I walked well enough to jettison my AFO and "go into the community" with a cane, but without a brace. After months of doing so, we were planning a trip to visit friends in Sweden, and I intended to travel AFO-less. Shortly before the trip, I wrote a post about shoes.

Posted 5th May 2011

As a shoe-lover, I have been discouraged buying shoes because of the need to buy 2 pairs to have 1 pair that fits. For our trip to Sweden, though, I need a pair of good walking shoes that I break in before heading there.

Yesterday, for the first time since the stroke, I went into my favorite shoe store in downtown Gloucester and bought one pair of shoes - black SAS walking shoes, size 7, plus some coiled laces so that I don't have to tie them. Then Patricia [a friend] and I fooled around trying to tie a shoelace one-handed. I've looked online for a way, but I don't like any of them [the methods pictured online] because not one looks like it was tied normally [the conventional way]. I like to keep my standards high despite my very good excuse not to. I finally figured out a way, but it would not untie easily, which defeats the purpose, right?

Anyway, I now have a comfy, good-looking pair of new shoes, and black, too, to finally match most of my clothes instead of wearing putty-colored, Velcro-close shoes with gray/black pants. There's that vanity again.

My issue with shoes continued. From the start, I had complained about not being able to wear cute shoes, and a dear friend gave me little black flats for Christmas just two months post-stroke, along with the sweetest note saying that she knew I'd soon be able to wear them. From that point on, I dreamed of dressing up and wearing those shoes, until I finally got a chance.

how did I forget the SHOES?"

Posted April 25, 2012

Two weekends ago, when Millie and I went to my
niece's shower in Philly, I got dressed up: long black
skirt; it was long enough to cover my Bioness leg cuff,
for which a friend criticized me - she said that I should
show off my L300 [Bioness leg brace I eventually got],
even flaunt it, because I have overcome more
adversity than most people face in a lifetime, and I
should be proud of myself despite the signs the stroke
left behind. PLUS I got to wear my never-yet-worn cute
shoes. A friend ... gave them to me the following
Christmas, along with a card that said something
along the lines of: "I know you'll ditch that brace and
wear regular shoes soon." The "soon" was not an
accurate prediction, but since then, I have had the goal
of wearing the lovely things: black flats decorated with
smooth silver and brass rivets on the surface. The
Bioness sensor clipped to the shoe, which has very
thin leather, which meant the clip had to go over
leather AND a rivet to be thick enough to clasp tight[ly]
enough to stay on. I was not able to handle that part
one-handed, so Tom was concerned I'd do it wrong
and end up tripping at the shower. To remedy that,
Tom called my younger sister the evening before the
shower to ask her to help me with it upon our arrival ...
I wore safe, sane shoes on the trip there, then
switched, with my sister's help, to the cute ones at the
restaurant. So, I FINALLY wore the cute shoes; there
were cuter ones [on other women] at the shower, but
all of them had heels too high for me to ever wear
again. That's fine by me because my feet always got
sore in high heels anyway. In fact, I also practiced
wearing the cute shoes at home without the Bioness
and I could manage that too, but didn't dare wear them

that way at the shower. I'll do it out in the community sometime "soon," though.

Is it safe to drive?

Driving is another important ADL. Being able to drive again is mostly dependent on your state's regulations, which range from a stroke having no effect on your driving status to needing to pass a driving test (written and/or road) again to get your license back. Look into your own state's regulations before assuming you can continue driving. If your state has not taken away your driving privileges, make sure you have some sort of evaluation to assess whether you are safe to drive.

When I had the stroke, I didn't know anything about driving after a brain injury. Massachusetts law – enforced by the Medical Affairs Division of the Registry of Motor Vehicles – stipulates that a driver's license must be suspended for 6 months following any incident of unconsciousness. I, in fact, was never unconscious – awake throughout the morning, entering the ER in Gloucester, and the coming and going of my symptoms. But there was no accommodation for that – a stroke is defined as accompanied by unconsciousness – so, I was required to not drive for at least six months, which was fine by me, but I didn't know that. My 6 months would be up May 12, 2010, but I didn't know I couldn't legally drive until then.

I pieced it together finally after applying for a handicap-parking placard. The application had to be signed by my physician explaining my physical need for one; he had to sign a statement with my condition (hemiparesis as a result of a stroke).

There was also a check-box asking whether I should have my driving evaluated in order to drive again. My PCP asked me whether he should check "yes," and I – not having a clue about the consequences of that – thought it sounded like a good, safe approach and said, "Yes."

Enormous mistake.

I received my placard, but the application contents started a cascade of letters from the RMV saying that my license was going to be revoked unless I took a road test within 30 days. Well, I was in no condition to take a test, so I ignored the letter. Ignoring each monthly letter, I made it through a few months, until I finally called the RMV to let them know it would be a while before I could take the test, and was told I had to call the Medical Division, (no, they could not give me the number and suggested I look for it online). The Medical Division told me that my license would be revoked unless I took the test within 30 days of the date of my most recent letter. No one told me that my other option was to voluntarily give up my license. Finally catching on that as long as I physically had the license, the RMV assumed I was still driving, which I was not supposed to do until I had my driving "evaluated," per my physician's suggestion.

Sometime around March (4 months after), I called RMV Medical Affairs and, after many transfers, found someone willing to talk to me about the situation. He said that if I turned in my license, they would "probably" stop the revocation process, and that I was better off trying to get my license back if I turned it in instead of if it were actually revoked. I asked him how to send it in. He said to mail it to the Medical Division (no, he didn't have the address, but was sure I could find it online) along with a letter of explanation, using the U.S. Postal Service. So, nervous that my license would be lost and untraceable, I did.

Then, although my husband was reluctant for me to try driving, I wanted to because I was not willing to have friends drive me to therapy and buy my groceries indefinitely; so for starters, I needed a permit to practice driving before taking the road competency test. Another call to the RMV landed me someone who told me that, because of my circumstances, I could not apply for a driving permit myself, but had to get a certified driving instructor to do so.

Seriously?

A local instructor said he had done it before and knew what to do. Within a week, my permit arrived in the mail. The process worked! All it took were a few dozen phone calls and persistence -- that is, time and tenacity. I had those.

I took a couple of driving lessons with the instructor, and while he was very helpful, he discouraged me from getting adaptive equipment for my car because that meant I would get a "restricted" license, which meant I could drive no other car – like my husband's, for example. And he thought I drove just fine without.

My next step was to pass an RMV-mandated eye test. I passed, then wrote the following blog entry.

RMV vision screening

Posted 10th June 2010

Yesterday's milestone was passing an eye test, one of two required tests to get my driver's license back. After applying for a handicap parking placard ... the Medical Affairs Division of the RMV informed me that in order to retain my license, I needed to pass a vision screening and a road competency test. I have not yet scheduled the road test, but hope to after taking some driving lessons with [a local] Driving School, which has applied for a temporary learner's permit for me to use during lessons with their instructors ...

As it is, I have not driven since Nov. 11, 2009, the day before the stroke and, although I drove for 26 [problem-free] years before that, I'm a bit nervous about being able to parallel park, etc. [one-handed] in a test situation - just as I was nervous that, when it came right down to it, I would fail the eye exam for some up-to-now-not-detected effect of the stroke, given that the medical personnel treating me since the stroke have relied on me noticing how I've been affected, when it came to eyesight - "Any double vision?" etc.

A month later (July 17, 2010) I had a seizure – the diagnosis was stroke-induced epilepsy – and the six-month no-driving clock started again.

Tick, tock.

Although I was eager to drive again, it took me nearly a year to muster the courage to actually schedule the test. Tom had little confidence in my ability to drive, and for a while refused to even go out driving with me on my permit, so I had few opportunities to practice. His fundamental complaint was that I was not aware of where the right side of my car was, which caused me to drive too close to the center line, which was one effect of the left-side neglect I experience.

Eventually, a vague sense of unease came over me whenever I thought about taking the test, so, I delayed.

Tick, tock.

Every time someone gave me a ride or I had to call a taxi, I lectured myself that I was being a coward: of course I could drive – think of all those years of accident-free driving anywhere and everywhere, including [once] on the left side of the street in England ... How could I not be able to drive the main streets in Lawrence during the test?

Adding to my anxiety, no one could tell me with assurance what was on the test. A couple of RMV employees told me hesitantly that a competency test was the same as a regular test. Seriously? Would I really have to pass the same test as a 17-year-old? 3-point turn? Parallel park?

One day Millie hassled me about not taking the test yet, and when I explained that I was anxious about it, that it was unknown, she had a terrific answer – to look at the first attempt to take the test as an attempt to gather information, to find out what the test was like. What would it matter if I failed? I'd still be dependent on others to drive me around, just as I was now, but I'd actually know what was on the test.

"Think of it like the PSAT," she said, "a practice test to let you know what the real thing will be like."

As soon as Tom okayed it, I scheduled the competency road test; I went to it with Tom, not my driving instructor.

Then on June 2, 2011, I blogged:

I failed the driving competency test

It was for a specific reason: I did not have adaptive equipment installed in my car to compensate for my one-handed driving. I need a knob on the steering wheel and a device that allows me to control the blinkers without taking my hand from the wheel. Now, if that's a requirement, why did every Mass. RMV employee (including in the Medical Division), ... and all my OTs and PTs I talked to not know that? All of them said I "could" get the equipment if I wanted to, not that it was required. How could none of them know? The closest was the suggestion that I have a driving evaluation by a post-stroke driving specialist to get his/her recommendations - it costs $300, which I didn't want to spend on someone who could say exactly what everyone else was saying. In fact, my driving instructor told me that the RMV "has to accommodate my disability," implying that if I use my right hand to do what my left hand is incapable of, I could still pass. My tester today, though, said that he really could not pass me because I MUST have the adaptive equipment ...

The good news, though, was that the tester told me that I was a very good, very safe driver and that if I'd had the adaptive equipment, I would have passed. He said the parallel parking was a little "iffy" because the car was not lined up straight at the end, but that was the only thing wrong. (I know, though, that I turned the wheels the wrong direction when he asked me to pretend I was parking on the side of a road on a hill, with a curb - I should have turned the wheel left, but I turned it to the right. So, he was a nice guy, which makes me believe that if he COULD have passed me, he would have.

I am very disappointed to not have my license now, but am happy to have followed Millie's advice to approach the first test as a PSAT to discover what the test is really like. So, here I am today, in the same situation I've been in for 18 months - not able to drive by myself. Except that now I know what's required ...

Now, if any of you are wondering why I never wrote about the upcoming driving test in this blog, I'll tell you: I didn't want to have to tell people that I failed. It was bad enough to fail, but the last thing I wanted was to have to admit it to absolutely everyone. And yet here we are. Post-stroke, there is no place for pride.

Once the RMV tester let me know what was required, I looked on the Internet to find someone who could install the adaptive equipment, but the nearest garage was at least an hour away; that discouraged me because Tom already has enough extra packed into his schedule because of me. Tom, though, looked online for the equipment, not an installer, and ordered both items. It didn't take long for him to install them, although the first clamps he used on the directional diverter didn't work well, and he experimented with other types. Then I had to practice using them.

The first issue with the knob was that it was in the way while I was *not* using it for a turn – even a slight curve in the road; so I decided to use it most of the time, not just when I needed it.

Having the directional control on the right side of the wheel, a couple of inches above the wiper controller, was more challenging. Thirty years of driving makes hitting a blinker or wiper automatic for anyone –- pre-stroke, I used to put the blinker on without a thought or a glance. Having it to the right, though, meant – and still means – that I first think that I'll need my blinker, then glance in that direction to ensure I'm going for the directional, not the wipers. And vice versa – when I need the wipers, I look to make sure I'm not heading toward the directional. Eventually, the movements will become second nature – there, I said it: I may *always* require adaptive equipment because I may not regain enough use of my arm/hand to drive without. Who cares? I'm not working hard on using my hand again in order to stop driving one-handed. Driving one-handed is fine, although it does make me anxious to not have certain motions automatic. That contributes to me not wanting to drive on highways – what if I had to switch lanes quickly and could not react fast enough to hit my blinker first? Of course, I can always use the excuse that I'm from Massachusetts, and we just don't use directionals.

As my six-month post-seizure date approached, I called the RMV and scheduled my second competency test. December 15 was the earliest date I could get, so I took it. It was not quite six months after having the seizure (July 17) but close enough for me:

progress today

After a very crappy, "this is too hard for me" day yesterday, the Universe made up for it today when I passed the driving competency test and came home with a driver's license!! ...

Once [my adaptive] equipment was in place, I practiced everything I needed to do correctly, signed up for another test and then waited 2 months to take it. .... It really was a high-stakes test because failure meant prolonging my dependence and reinforcing my what-is-called "learned helplessness," which develops when someone doesn't do tasks for so long that the ability goes away or never develops. For example, if someone else had been dressing me for the past 2 years, I would not know how to dress myself. Ditto for walking, showering, etc.

I am feeling now the same - or similar - sense of freedom and possibility I felt when I first got my license at 17!

Bottom-line: I took the test, I passed it, and I walked out of the RMV with a temporary paper license that meant I could drive anywhere, anytime, but needed to be driving a car with (1) adaptive equipment and (2) an automatic transmission.

Since that day, my drives have been conservative: I sometimes go back roads to avoid one particular rotary. For a long time, I didn't spend more than 30 minutes on Route 128, with scary, fast-moving (75 mph) strings of cars, using short entry ramps and driven by brazen self-absorbed drivers talking on cell phones. Six months later (on May 18, 2012), when I wrote the following entry, not much had changed ...

Driving Route 128

My husband was very concerned about me getting my license back because he was convinced that I'd get in an accident ... Finally, he agreed it would be acceptable, as long as: (1) I stayed in Gloucester (2) I did not drive at night or in bad weather (3) I did not drive on highways and (4) I avoided the highway portion of Route 128 as much as I could. I agreed, thinking that they would be temporary restrictions and I would eventually be able to [drive where I wanted]... Yesterday, though, I ventured out [beyond the imposed boundaries] ... [I had an] appointment yesterday at 10:30 a.m. I set out at 9:30 for what Google maps said would be a 30-minute drive. ... Fortunately, the shop was just a right turn at the end of the ramp and an immediate right into a plaza.. Easy, with no possibility of getting lost. No trouble at all - except for having 30 minutes to kill because I was so early. The return trip was just as uneventful and even included merging into oncoming traffic to get on 128 ... Bottom line [is that] I drove 30 minutes on 128 twice yesterday and NOTHING bad happened. ...

Now, nearly 5 years post-stroke, as I write this book, I have actually driven for two two-hour stretches, on lightly traveled highways in good weather. It was a significant jump from my previous record of 45-minute drives. But I did it because I had a significant goal – driving myself back to the newspaper office where I used to work. And I drove myself there for the first time post-stroke, not being driven or taking the commuter rail. I took the long way – or one of the long ways. And I drove myself home too, at the end of my visit there. That's 4 hours of driving in a single day.

Being able to drive again was a short-term goal immediately after the stroke, but, like most parts of recovery, it ended up taking far more calendar time than I expected – or planned.

That's also been the case for other short-term goals – Four years later and there are many not-recovered "short-term goals." But, to drive, I persevered and got there – eventually.

Traveling

By foot

Mobility is a top priority for stroke survivors. Nothing emphasizes a survivor's dependence as much as not being able to get around. For me, immediately after the stroke, there was getting from a wheelchair to my feet (called "sit-to-stand," a primary focus of a PT) and then learning to get my affected foot forward in a step-like fashion.

In the beginning, wearing an AFO, I used a couple of techniques to take steps: raising myself to the toes of my unaffected foot so that I could swing my other foot straight forward, just clearing the floor; and swinging my affected leg out so that my foot traveled in a clockwise arc from back to front, which is called circumducting, and it is the way a stroke survivor's muscles work together (called synergy) trying to get the job done after brain damage prevents the coordination of individual muscles. I used circumduction (swinging my foot in an arc, back to front) for years even though each of my PT's try to teach me how to walk without doing so. The correct way is to engage my hamstring to bend my knee, my quads to lift my knee, then swing my foot forward while keeping my toes raised. It took me 3.5 years of walking to be able to control my hamstring (my weakest link, according to my physiatrist), so that's really when I could start improving my gait. My hamstring is still not strong enough to bend my knee as far as it should in order to take an approximately correct step.

By car

Although I eventually got my driver's license back, I had many places to go before that, and we devised a range of solutions. At first, I had two dear friends who insisted on – and persisted at – taking me to weekly PT and OT sessions. I had my first year of outpatient therapy at a clinic a half-hour from home, OT and PT scheduled back-to-back on Tuesday and Friday afternoons. One friend spent my two-hour sessions reading in the waiting room on Tuesdays, and the other visited her grandchildren in the same town on Fridays. That lasted 9 months, until my insurance-allowed visits were used up.

By taxi

When I first needed to go on short trips and didn't want to inconvenience a friend, I took a cab.

When I was newly disabled, there was a new cab company in Gloucester, written up in the local paper. So the first time I took a cab, I decided to support the new business, and called that company.

I explained that I was disabled, so although I would be near the door waiting, it would take me some time to come out to the car, and could the driver please stop at the door at the left-hand end of the house?

As it turned out, the driver was from one of the old-time Gloucester families. He knocked, then came into the house to see if he could help me. We leave our door unlocked because so many people come by to say, "hi," deliver dinner, and otherwise help out, but it takes me so long to get to the door, it's better for friends to just enter. The driver coming in surprised me, though. I expected a honk, and instead, there was a stranger in my kitchen. He was friendly and moved to take my arm, but I explained that I would be fine by myself, although opening and holding the storm door would be a big help.

He insisted on me sitting in the front passenger seat and got me to my destination safely. Because he came around to open my car door when we got there, it was easy to pay him. I knew the fee, and used a single $10 bill I had clenched in my fist so that I didn't have to fumble with multiple bills, and told him to keep the change. All to make it easier.

Other cab rides didn't go as easily.

When I used to go to Mass. General for OT, I tried to have cash in the correct amount for each leg of the trip: train, cab, appointment, then cab followed by train. One morning, though, we were short on cash. Although Tom had told me that cabs take credit cards, I was too nervous to rely on that. What if I got into a cab without a card reader?

As it turned out, I worried the whole train ride about not having the cash for the cab, but when I got into one by the Bobby Orr statue outside of North Station, it had the card reader right there in front of me. When we got to the hospital, I explained that I had never used credit in a cab before, so he verbally walked me through the instructions. Everything went fine. I relaxed, content that I could handle payment after the cab ride back to North Station.

At North Station on my return trip, though, I swiped my card, but couldn't get the reader (or my card) to work. After a dozen or so attempts, I explained that I couldn't figure out how to use it. Instead of verbal instructions, the driver popped out of his seat and got in the back seat next to me. He swiped my card, then proceeded through the process, leaning across my lap to see the screen.

When he got to the tip entry, he looked at me, "Tip?"

How awkward is that? I felt I had no choice – there he was taking the time to fix this for me *and* was watching. What else do you do when the service person is watching you commit to the tip? I told him a *very* generous amount, and he finished up the transaction. Then he jumped out, went around the car, opened my door, and helped me out.

My physiatrist's office was at the old location of Spaulding Rehab Hospital in Boston, a 15-minute walk from North Station, the final destination of the commuter rail from Gloucester. To get there, either Tom drove me, or I took a cab from my house to the Gloucester train station, took the one-hour train ride, disembarked at North Station, and walked to the hospital. I preferred taking the train over Tom taking off the day to drive me there. Taking the train was a step in my quest for independence.

By train

Boarding the train always makes me nervous that the train would start moving before I was seated; disembarking made me nervous because I couldn't stand up until the train stopped completely, and I am always anxious the train will leave the station before I make it to the exit. In both cases on the train home to Gloucester, I have to walk as fast as possible to make it to either the seat or the door before the train starts off; and I am very slow, which increases my insecurity.

As a result, I have sometimes liked to draw attention to myself so that the staff in my car would know I was disabled and needed extra time. I have often asked for the metal plate be put down that covered the gap between the platform and the train, mostly because my fear of heights makes the gap particularly deep and scary, but also to communicate that I am disabled and needed special consideration.

At North Station, in addition to having to board, I have to walk on the platform the entire length of the train because the car with a doorway that opened even with platform height (meaning I don't have to go up or down the train stairs, which are much too steep for me) is at the end farthest from the station. The first time I returned home by train, I timed my walk to the correct car, and it took me 20 minutes. After that, I would ask early at the help desk what track the Gloucester (Rockport) train would use (so that I could get a head start) and got the same answer: "We won't know that until 10 minutes before departure. That's when we announce it. You'll have to wait until we announce it."

Now, I knew that could not possibly be true, so I stated the obvious:

"As you can see, I walk very slowly – in fact it takes me 20 minutes to walk to the correct car because I have to go to the very first car. Which means the train will leave 10 minutes late. If I can get a 10-minute head start, I'll be able to board when the other passengers do, and the train can leave on time."

"I'm sorry, but we don't know which track until the train's nearly here."

"Surely someone here knows which track the Gloucester train will be on."

"But we can't guarantee which track it will be, and you don't want to be started down one track, then have to turn around and have to walk all the way back and down the correct one. Right?"

It was obviously time for the big guns, the "disabled card," referring to the Americans With disabilities Act:

"Look, I'm disabled. You have to accommodate me. How are you going to do that?"

He picked up the phone and pressed the right buttons. After deflecting a lot of crap on the other end of the line, he looked at me.

"You want the Rockport train, right?"

I nodded.

"Track 2."

Someone really did already know. "Thank you so much. I appreciate your help."

And I was able to board and take a seat in the front car before the train left the station.

From that point on, the same staff member was at the help desk every time I was heading home from Mass General. As I would approach his window, he would give me a big smile and hold up his fingers indicating the track number (it was always track 1, 2, or 3) and mouth, "Rockport?"

I would nod, smile and mouth, "Thank you."

Eventually, I got my walking time down to 10 minutes, and, like everyone else, would wait for the general announcement of the track number. That meant other passengers swarmed around me, leaving me to struggle along the last couple of cars with other disabled people, the elderly, parents with strollers, and 20-somethings with bicycles, all who needed an exit level with the platform.

By plane

A job lured our son to California two years ago. Before that, he lived in Manhattan for a few years. Manhattan is a five-hour drive from here, while California's a five-hour flight; he claims that's equivalent, and even tried to prove it by showing up at home for a family reunion the weekend after he moved west. Show-off.

As he sauntered up to me at the reunion, a complete surprise, arms spread to give me a bear hug, I was crying.

"You're making me cry," I said as he gave me that hug.

"That was my goal," he said, "and to show you that California's not that far away.

He's wrong, though -- for me, a five-hour trip by car makes very few demands on me. Tom drives, I sit with the dog on my lap, the back seat has a bag of snacks, the cup holder has a bottle of water, and everything I will need or want is in the trunk. I don't have to carry anything at any point.

Flying five hours is different ...

Traveling

Posted 19th December 2012

We - my husband, daughter and I - are going to California (Santa Monica) to visit our son and his fiancée for Christmas. Another trip through security [my first experience was flying to Boulder for a friend's son's wedding] holding my left hand as far as my right hand can raise it in the X-ray machine; having my entire body (all my clothing, really) and electronic gear swabbed and tested for explosives; giving up my cane to walk through the metal detector; standing on a two-foot square for a full-body search. On our last flight, a security person chided me for leaving a tissue in my back pocket ... revealed by the search even though she had TOLD me to empty my pockets; I pulled it out and handed it to her, and she went to get a trash can, watching me the whole time. Seriously? What was I going to do with a used tissue if she turned her back to me? I can understand why she didn't want to touch it, but watching me while she walked sideways to get the can and carry it to me? What happened to profiling? I am doing something a little differently this time, compared to our last flight (to Boulder): I am going to cooperate with my husband and use a WHEELCHAIR. He always frets because I walk so slowly, but I hate taking the easy way out. My recovery is all about challenging myself, so why wouldn't I walk? To please Tom. He puts up with enough annoyance caused by me; it's the least I can do, I think. And in February, I'm going BY MYSELF to visit a friend who spends the winter in Florida. Tom will accompany me to the airport and ensure I get through security okay, and Lisa will pick me up at the other end. Wheelchairs at both ends. One good thing about wheelchairs at the airport is that they come with a driver, someone to push and steer, and knows what line to go to, plus gets to cut every line. In fact, when Tom once took over for a driver at Logan, he had to go through a 50-point check before I was handed over. I am afraid to travel by air all alone. I know I'll be well taken care of, but I'm still nervous about it.

While my experiences flying haven't been awful, I did find security an annoyance and intrusion, humiliating even, that an obviously disabled woman has to, fundamentally, prove she's not trying to carry on a banned item. I was instructed to hold my hands over my head – I couldn't. I was asked to get out of the airline's wheelchair and walk without my cane through the metal detector; without my cane because it was off in an adjacent line getting patted down. *Plus* I had to get out of the wheelchair again and stand, feet apart, for a few minutes for my own pat-down, including – time after time – being told that the searcher was going to touch my private areas with the backs of her gloved hands. Seriously? As if I cared at that point.

When we've made reservations, we've always managed to get me an aisle seat so that I won't disturb anyone climbing out to go to the restroom every hour or so.

At our previous home, we made wonderful friends who were from Sweden. In 2001, after raising their two children here (a son and daughter the same ages as our own), they returned home to Stockholm. Since then we've wanted to visit them there, but didn't until 18 months after I had the stroke.

At home I was going completely without an AFO, or any brace, but used a cane. I planned to see Sweden the same way. The one concession I made was, as insurance, to take the AFO "just in case" something happened and I needed it while we were there. I wore it rather than packing it because of luggage space. Overall, I was fine going without it.

Sweden

Posted 17th May 2011

Who knew that the king's palace in Stockholm is surrounded by every kind of cobblestone in the world? When we went there yesterday, I expected smooth surfaces. Instead, there were small round cobbles, large round and small and large flat square and rectangular ones. Plus hundreds of [shallow] steps inside, from the formerly rat-infested cellar up to the gilt-pillar room where citizens used to receive awards from the king. We took a bus tour of the city, too, so we were not walking the entire day. I wore my small black Velcro ankle brace, which I have not previously successfully used on uneven surfaces. More progress.

Another accomplishment for me was making my way through Central Station [in Stockholm] during rush hour in order to take the commuter train back to Sigtuna, where we are staying. Although there were plenty of opportunities to be jostled, I managed to make my way through the crowd, my friend Kerstin setting a pick and Tom at my back. Millie often scouted ahead to find restrooms, stairways, elevators and entrances as needed.

Obviously, I need a lot of support when traveling.

Eventually, I was adept enough at flying that I managed to fly by myself to Florida and back.

Traveling without a keeper

Posted 12th January 2013

I usually get a lot of help - especially when I travel. Since having the stroke, Tom and I (and sometimes Millie) have flown to Sweden, California and Philadelphia [plus Boulder, Col.] ... I have a dear friend who spends a couple of months every winter in Florida. This year it's January and February. She rents a two-bedroom condo in Jupiter, so invites friends and family to visit. Last week I flew south to stay for a long weekend - Thursday to Monday. Tom agreed to me going, despite the fact I would be traveling alone. Oh, imagine that: Barb loose in the world. The plan that made him comfortable was him accompanying me to the gate (which he was allowed to do because wheel-chaired people can have someone stay with them until boarding) and Lisa meeting me at baggage claim in the West Palm airport. His greatest worry was, seriously, how Turbo would fare in my absence. No worries about me, not really. Imagine the scene: Again everyone did everything for me, Tom pulled my suitcase to check-in, while the wheelchair driver swooshed us to the fast line, bypassed the line at security, stopped me at the bathroom, and got me to the gate just as pre-boarding started (no time for Tom to get me coffee). The driver had my boarding pass and swooshed me right down the jetway. I was in - the logistics were almost halfway completed. On the other end, a wheelchair met me at the exit door of the plane, swooshed me to baggage claim, found my bag, then left me and the bag to meet Lisa, who dumped my bag in the back of her car and took us to Starbucks. My return is 3 days away, and I imagine it will be the same, but in reverse. Bottom line: traveling alone was not that different from going with someone. I still had little to do except answer security questions and indicate when I wanted to use the restroom. And Turbo is fine. PLUS, I will have been to Jupiter and back.

Steps in My Own Recovery

For me, recovery has fallen into several categories: cognitive, physical (arm/hand and leg), and emotional. As stroke survivors go, I am fortunate. Not only did I live, the stroke I had was on the right side of my brain, which means I lost the use of my left side, which is my non-dominant side. Plus it means that my language center (located in the left side of my brain) was not affected. Otherwise, it could have resulted in something called aphasia, which leaves some survivors with a range of language problems, from being unable to recognize written characters, read and/or speak to not being able to retrieve the desired word while speaking/writing.

Whichever side a stroke survivor loses, there is always hope for improvement – although maybe not complete recovery - for all of us. Some of the recovery can be regaining the lost ability, while other times it can be through gaining compensatory abilities that allow us to do a lost activity, but in a different way. An example of the former would be to recover an affected dominant hand to the point of being able to write a signature, while another solution is for a non-dominant hand to "learn" to sign a name. Each survivor gets to choose an approach acceptable for him/her – either attempting to do something the way they did it pre-stroke, or compensating by finding a different way to do it.

Personally, I am so goal-oriented that I just want to get the task done, whatever way I can..

My first outpatient OT consisted of working on devising ways for me to complete ADL's. This included taking a shower by myself, which means figuring out how to stay safe, using soap, opening shampoo bottles, and keeping dry towels dry, which all require more ingenuity than it appears; getting dressed; cooking; washing dishes; and getting into cars, for example. These are, of course, all practical acts that enable a survivor to be responsible for standard participation in life. At my first session with my first OT, she asked me if I wanted to learn to tie my sneakers one-handed. Of course I said no thanks, because I was convinced that any day, I would be using my affected hand and tying my shoes with both hands. Now, four-and-a-half years later, I am still wearing the spring-shaped elastic laces that little kids wear. I rejected Velcro closures long ago because of a personal vendetta against the product. The elastic laces come in black for my walking shoes, white for my sneakers, and a rainbow of bright colors I have to make work for the rest, although I live in my walking shoes and sneakers, so that's a moot point.

One of the points I want to make is that uncertainty is part of life. Four years ago I planned on being able to use both hands to tie my shoes any minute, but I was wrong. Determination can result in the accomplishment of many goals, but there's no seeing into the future. All of us are working into an unknown future. Hard work, not force of will, will get us – all of us, not just stroke survivors – to achieve our goals.

After seeing the MRI of my post-stroke brain, I thought of a visual analogy describing my injury: my skull had been sawed open at the top (like a jack-o-lantern) and someone had used an ice cream scoop to remove a third of my brain, put it in a blender and then poured it back into my skull - a thick pink (or would it be gray?) milkshake of lumpy liquefied brain matter. That analogy came to my defense, always internally, whenever I did something stupid. What

86

did I expect from myself after one-third of my brain had been pureed? Of course I had "brain fog."

Now I know, though, that it would have been helpful had my physiatrist (1) identified which parts were dead and which were in the penumbra of the stroke (a stunned portion that could be expected to possibly spontaneously recover or recover by dint of hard work) and (2) identified which parts of my brain (functionally – for example, the motor cortex) were in a dead area (expected to never recover) so that to recover the function lost, I would have to get another part of my brain to take over that function (also by dint of hard work, not spontaneously)

Thank God for the neuroplasticity of the brain – a recent understanding that the brain is changeable and that areas of it can be trained to perform new tasks. To me, this means that although I have lost forever the area of my brain that made my left hand respond to my thoughts, I need to inspire a different area to do it instead. Despite neuroplasticity, convincing any part of the brain to do something it has never done is a profoundly difficult thing that may take hundreds of thousands, or even millions, of repetitions (attempts to perform the action, even without successfully using the muscle), as I wrote about in this blog entry:

I did WHAT?

Posted 11th March 2013

Let's do the math: In the stroke community, one topic is about how many repetitions are required to result in rewiring our brain to communicate with a distant muscle no longer connected to its original boss in our brain. We exercise aerobically to optimize neurogenesis [the creation of new brain cells] and we try repeatedly to perform the feat we want to accomplish. How many times do we have to repeat it? Two weeks ago, I had the thrilling success of using my left biceps femoris, semitendinosus, and semimembranosus muscles ([together a.k.a. the hamstring, which makes a knee bend] for the first time post-stroke. Out of curiosity, I decided to answer the "How many repetitions does it take?" question: In addition to all the muscle-specific exercises demanded of me by my therapists over the years and many uses of the hamstring Nautilus equipment at the Y, along with attempting to raise my knee (and use my hamstring) every step up on stairs, plus electrical stimulation, and taking nearly-daily walks – all performed over a span of the 3.5 years since having a stroke – I have also WALKED. By that I mean daily incidental walking (incidental to life, with at least a short conventional walk), and taking each step, I tried to get my hamstring to bend my knee. When I got my new Bioness [an electronic leg brace], I turned in my "trial" unit and it turned out to have saved all my daily walking data, which ranged from a low of 2,500 to a high of 5,000 or 6,000. ... [at a minimum, I walked ... 2,000 steps per day over 3.5 years]. Although a person with a proper gait is advised to walk at least 10,000 steps/day, I don't think 2,000 for me is shoddy. I have done that every day for 3.5 years, (365 x 3.5 x 2,000 = 2,555,000). That is two-and-a-half MILLION attempts to use my hamstring. It is a daunting number, but it works out to about 170 attempts per hour for a 12-hour day (7 a.m. to 7 p.m.) or 3 times/minute during everyday life, which doesn't seem too hard to do. Got to focus on these fingers. [But, of course, it did take 3.5 years and persistence.]

I don't want that number to discourage anyone, but rather to set the bar so that discouragement doesn't come with a lack of results, even after very hard work. There is a long way to go, yes, but calendar time goes by rapidly anyway, so you may as well use the time to progress, even little by little. You will see results, no matter where you want to focus. And where you focus is your choice:

My future: arm vs. leg

Posted 22nd September 2012

Yesterday I had the pleasure of a visit from two old friends - one ... had a stroke 31 years ago, long before I met her. ... Of course, as soon as they arrived, I assessed the extent of recovery of the stroke survivor, something I'll bet she was doing about me too. We were similar, although she'd had a stroke on the left side of her brain, which had impaired her speech, something that appeared to me to be fine, although she said she still struggles with talking and speaks much more slowly than she used to. Our differences: as I said, the side of her impairment; her arm shows much more spasticity than mine, hugged in close to her chest, hand clenched; her leg, though, behaves well enough in her AFO that she can walk around the community without a cane. For a long set of stairs (not a single or even two steps in a row), she seems to need a rail, wall or arm to descend, while I still put too much of my weight on my cane or rail to descend even

90

one step without. While I dream of (i.e., imagine) going into the community - and even outside - cane-less, I wouldn't dream (i.e., think) of doing that; I rely too much on it. Another difference: she was 37 when the stroke struck. Going cane-less has the tremendous advantage of being able to carry objects. I would be able to fly somewhere and pull my own suitcase, even if I were alone; I would be able to carry my own plate at a buffet. At home, I'm okay with all this because I can walk short distances without my cane and so, carry something with me. This morning I was pondering which would be better: to be able to go cane-less or to use my left hand? I decided on cane-less because my friend could do so much more than I could; she could nearly blend in with everyone else. When I walked into the restaurant we chose, the staff was attentive and even held open the restroom door for me; as we wove through the tables, diners and wait staff moved out of the way of me and my cane. There was no special treatment for my friend because she didn't need it. I don't mind standing out; I'm actually on a crusade to be as visible as I can be so that people know what a stroke survivor looks like. Now if I look into the future - which is my MO - if, in 28 years from now, I can do as much as my friend, I'm okay with that. And I'll have had 28 more years of working on getting this frigging hand to work.

Rehabbing arm/hand

Someone once communicated a novel (to me) concept: a hand is a tool, and an arm is a delivery method to get the tool where we want to use it. Given that point of view and the fact that I want to resume rowing, I concluded that getting the tool fixed was the more important task, and I have focused on that - holding an oar.

Conventional "wisdom" is that hemiparesis recovery proceeds from the trunk, down the extremity, shoulder to fingers, and hip to toes. But it seemed that it would be easier for my arm to come along if the hand were useful enough to keep the far end in place. Of course, as usual, I did what I thought was best – hand first. Given that I have little use of either my arm (except for my shoulder) or hand right now, nearly five years out, I don't have an opinion about whether I have taken the correct approach. Even now, though, if I could get my hand to grasp an oar or the handle of my rowing machine, I am convinced that my fledgling biceps and triceps could get in the game. And I continue on under that belief.

Initially, my hand and arm were flaccid and impossible for me to move – either open or close my hand or move my arm in any direction. To move either my left arm or hand, I used my right, reaching over and positioning it where I wanted it, usually out of the way of something, like a seatbelt or the arm on a chair.

My first progress in that area was two months after the stroke:

fingers on my recalcitrant hand

Posted 10th January 2010

Today's topic was an easy decision: watching the Patriots [living northeast of Boston, I have no choice re a favorite team] today (AFC wild-card game against Baltimore), I gripped my left hand with my right in an attempt to warm up the left. While gripping it, my left hand responded by gripping back. When that happened, I could feel which muscles were working, so I pulled my right hand back and used it to straighten out the fingers on my left hand, then willed those muscles to contract again - and the fingers on my left hand curled toward my left palm! It's not that I successfully made a fist or anything like that - it was more like the fingers went from being straight to being bent at a right angle. It's great progress because I see it as the first step in being able to [use it].

I found out later that my grip at that time was probably resulting from the onset of spasticity, the involuntary contraction, of a predictable set of muscles. Spasticity in the upper extremity causes the classic post-stroke arm position: the hand is fisted and the arm hugged in tight against the body. Specifically, fingers are contracted into a fist, wrist is flexed, forearm is pronated (palm face-down) and biceps are contracted (bending the arm at the elbow). While mild spasticity can look like ability (as in my blog entry above), two problems are that, (1) the muscles opposing the spastic ones are weak (for example, the finger extensors are flaccid, while the finger flexors are contracted into a fist) and (2) there's no brain-to-muscle connection. It's challenging to get the weak muscles to overcome the spastic muscles, delaying recovery. Left to their own devices, a hand immobilized into a fist will eventually lose enough cells in the adjacent inner soft tissue that it will never be able to return to its intended relaxed state, and the fingers will not straighten, even passively (by someone else).

94

This makes it imperative that I keep my spastic muscles (all of them, not just those controlling the hand) stretched. Post-stroke, but before spasticity began, my arm and hand were flaccid and motionless. According to the Brunnstrom theory of recovery phases, from flaccid (stage 1) to spastic (stage 2) is a step toward recovering control of your affected muscles/movements as you overcome spasticity. If you are interested in recovery stages per Brunnstrom, I suggest you find an online reference, to help you figure out where you are versus how you'll reach your goal. It's information I didn't learn about until at least 6 months post-stroke, but it answered a lot of my previous questions, questions my medical team couldn't (or wouldn't) answer. Again, you must do your own research to find out both factual information about your situation *and* treatment options; unless, of course, you find the rare medical team that knows all the information you could use and can effectively communicate it to you.

While initially post-stroke, I could find no data about the likelihood of my recovery, I wrote a blog entry after I ran into this interesting information, which ends up being not bad news at all, almost a year post-stroke:

bad news from an AHA study

15th October 2010

A stroke recovery website sent me this today:

"According to a major study by the American Heart Association, 44% percent of stroke survivors say that arm movement is their most common physical challenge. Only 5% of adult stroke survivors regain full arm function and 20% regain no functional use."

It's the final statement that bothers me. I have no intention of being part of that 20% statistic - what it means to me is that 80% regain some functional use - and that gives me more than a 50-50 chance; in fact, it's nearly assured. Not bad odds, if you ask me. Of course, the key statistic is the mere 5% that recover fully - something I have planned on all along. Can I manage to be part of that 5%?

This, in fact, is the kind of data I wanted when I first had the stroke, but no one could provide the info to me. How can that be when something like 6 million Americans have survived strokes and many have lasting effects [disabilities]? Think of the numbers that are available for statistical analysis: how could no one have [compiled] the statistics until now? To me, it seems like the first step in helping someone cope with what has happened to him/her.

I know that when I was in the rehab hospital, all the medical personnel were optimistic about me regaining all previous function, mostly because I was "young." Young for having a stroke, anyway [although since then I've earned that in utero babies have strokes, and I've met 20- and 30-somethings who have had them too. That [the "young" comment] has bolstered my hope throughout this ordeal - to think of myself as young enough to beat this thing. Plus I'm strong, stubborn, persistent, hard-working, not easily discouraged, and I have an enormous amount of support. "If anyone can recover, it would be me," has been what my head and my heart have been telling me all along. Delusional, you might call me, but I like to think not.

In fact, when I first started OT after getting out of the rehab hospital, my attitude was that I didn't need to learn to do anything else [other than self-care] one-handed because I wasn't going to be one-handed for very much longer. And here it is, my one-year anniversary [Nov.12] approaching. If anyone had told me that I was going to be one-handed and not driving (related only because they are hugely significant losses) a year after the stroke, I would not have believed them at all. So, maybe getting all that data shortly after the stroke would not have been helpful - knowing me, I would have dismissed it and remained optimistic."

Ever since reading that AHA information, I have been pleasantly surprised and proud of myself to see any progress by my upper extremity, as shown by this entry two months later:

and the recalcitrant arm moves!!!

Posted December 2010

Hooray!!! This morning in the wee hours (3:30), while I was lying on my back in bed, with my left arm resting across my torso, I tried pulling my toes up and flexing my foot, which I continuously try while I'm in my bed. As Dean [Reinke, the most knowledgeable stroke survivor I know online] ... said, recovery is a 24/7 job. Then [my attention] moved to my hand and I gripped my hand into a fist as tightly as I can, then on to trying to lift my arm, which actually happened! I lifted my arm about 2 inches off my torso and then had it move my hand a couple inches to the right. I found it miraculous and tried again, just to be sure - and it happened again. Given that stroke survivors often have a problem with proprioception (the ability to tell where their limbs are in space) and that I often "feel" my arm, legs, fingers and toes "doing" the things I want them to and am trying to communicate to them, I doubted that it was true. In the dark, I couldn't look to verify, which is what I normally do, so I woke up Tom (yes, he IS a saint) and asked him to feel whether my arm was moving. I did it again with him touching me and he said, "Yes, you're moving it!"

What a relief that all my work is not in vain! :)"

By April 2010, my arm was improving a bit, although sometimes it wasn't obvious:

the small yellow ball

Posted 16th April 2010

Success today took the form of a small yellow ball at occupational therapy. As I was lying down, OT Stephanie had me put my hands on either side of it and push it toward the ceiling until both arms were fully extended, then lower it to my chest and/or abdomen, then up again. To do it, I recruited every arm muscle I could remember looking at in Dr. Netter's atlas of human anatomy. Up, down, 10 times, then 10 more. When she asked me how that felt, I said, "Like my right arm was doing most of the work."

"Your left arm was working, too, though, or it would have flopped back down, which it didn't," she said. "How did it feel?"

It occurred to me that my left arm - that stupid recalcitrant one - had finally successfully accomplished something. Instead of my OT asking me to do something and having my left arm fail, my arm did it! How did that make me feel? I burst into tears; she patted me on the shoulder and asked me whether I was getting any counseling to help me with my ordeal. I said no, because I thought I was all right dealing with the whole thing. Given, though, how fragile I have become for being such a strong person, she had a good point and I'm thinking that next week I'll look into my counseling options.

As time went by and my disappointment in my arm/hand progress grew – time spent on exercises and calendar time rushing by - I talked to my PT [at the time] about using a Saebo Reach, an ingenious product designed to use springs to straighten out a patient's fingers after grasping a ball. With the Saebo on, I would flex my fingers to pick up a Nerf-like ball, pivot at my shoulder so that my hand was over a washbasin on a table, then relax my fingers. The springs would take over then and straighten my fingers so that the ball fell into the basin. Six balls moved one way, six the opposite way, repeat for an hour twice a day. It added up to a lot of balls – and a lot of time.

Here is my report about a successful session with my Saebo.

to my chin

Posted 13th September 2011

One of the exercises my Saebo OT gave me at my last session with her was to, using the Saebo, pick up a ball from in front of me, touch my chin with it and then drop it in a bucket, also in front of me, but a little to the right. I am to do it as many times as I can in 45 minutes. The first time I did it, I could strain every muscle (including my toes) without my hand making it very far up; it was 45 minutes of never getting anywhere near my chin. I progressed, though, so that in the second session, I brought the ball up to my waist; another 45 minutes of failing in my task.

Two days ago, I got closer to my chin and called Tom into the room to witness it; he estimated it was about 10 inches below my chin ... I reliably got the ball to ... what I measured as 8 inches! ... And I hope to [get within 6 inches] this afternoon. The exercise is to improve my elbow flexion, which will help me with other exercises.

After spending 7 months using the Saebo and seeing no functional improvement (yes, my OT kept measuring increasing range of motion in my elbow, but nothing resulted that I would call functional), I decided to stop using it, decided that I could spend my time more productively. So I stopped, and it's been packed in my closet since then. Overlapping with my other exercises, I joined a challenge at the Y in order to use the Nautilus equipment for my legs and abs; the organized challenge was to run/bike/swim 100 miles. The staff approved me walking/stationary biking/rowing machine instead. I tracked my progress using stickers on a grid in the gym.

Every once in a while, I'd have a break-through, something that captivated me into believing I'd get to the final recovery finish line after all, despite my failure to see progress:

my biceps

Posted 20th July 2012

Six months ago when I saw my physiatrist, he asked me if I could touch my chin. I said "No," then proceeded to try. Trying consisted of swinging my arm - synergy [inappropriate muscles jumping in to help] at work - so that my fist approached my chin. From the doctor's angle, it looked as though there was contact, but there really wasn't. Last week, he asked again, so I tried again, again swinging my arm, but this time making contact for real. Now - yesterday and today - I can actually bend my arm and move my hand up and touch my chin - my biceps in action, separately from all her buddies who've been jumping in and helping out. Progress! About 6 months post-stroke, I complained to [one] of my early OTs that my upper arm was hurting. She prodded around to locate the [painful] spot and then grinned as she told me that it was my "tiny biceps trying to grow stronger," that I had worked it enough to make it sore. Through disuse after the stroke, all the muscles on my left side atrophied. From that tiny sore muscle to being strong enough to bend my elbow and raise my forearm and hand to my chin is progress I'm proud of.

unreproducible thumb movement

Posted 11th August 2011

At 6 this morning, while sitting in bed drinking coffee, I swear I saw my thumb straighten! I then flexed it toward my palm and tried again, but could not reproduce the motion since then - and, yes, I HAVE been trying. Long ago, one of my OTs told me, after I attempted raising my shoulder 10 times, that my affected muscles tend to tire after three repetitions of a movement, and I suspect that the first time is the most tiring. I plan to spend the day periodically trying to straighten my thumb again and having Patricia (a friend helping me with my rehab) witness it straight ...

On occasion, my wonderful OT was out sick; sometimes a great one filled in, sometimes not-so-great. It was always hard for me to have a sub. There I am, raring to go, and the OT is reading my chart and trying to figure out what to do with me. The week I hit 10 miles on the Y challenge, 2 years post-stroke, I wrote this:

101

forearm pronation

Posted 22nd February 2011

A couple of weeks ago, a substitute OT told me that in order to row [a gig boat], I would have to be able to pronate (rotate from palm up to palm down) 100% of the time; this was after I told her I could look at my watch "on occasion." So, I added that capability to my Excel spreadsheet, where I keep track of daily progress in certain tasks. When I started, I could do it 4 times out of 10 attempts; two days ago, I did it 10 out of 10 and again this morning. It's never pretty, never held out in front of my torso (always resting against it or on my lap), never anything like when my right hand does it - so I suppose that means I continue practicing every day. [This is one of the exercises that dropped out of my arsenal along the way, forgotten, like many other things]...

Also, using my elbow splint during my morning arm exercises [done lying in bed before getting up], I was able to slowly lift and lower my arm from resting next to my body to pointing toward the ceiling 10 times without my right arm helping. And I did my leg exercises without any help from Tom, despite his frequent offer to help whenever my form was bad; my form will get better, though, and he will be able to go back to going to work very early.

At times, I had wonderful therapists who were experienced, knowledgeable, encouraging, always on my side, and genuinely helpful; but that was not always the case. Based on my experiences, I now make sure I respect and admire my therapists, and verify that they keep up-to-date on current therapies.

During one several-months period of therapy, I had a not-so-great OT. She had *never* worked with a stroke survivor, but was local, which was a big plus. When I requested an OT with more relevant experience, the response was that the clinic had no OT with any stroke survivor experience; one OT even said, "An arm is an arm." As an example of her "not-so-greatness," she once gave me an exercise to do that I could not actually do. She had me try a dozen times (with her watching) to swipe a rag across a counter using a sweeping motion, with a cloth under my forearm to reduce friction. I could not do it, which she clearly saw.

"How many reps, and how many times a day?" I asked, lamb to the slaughter.

"100 times every hour." I think she was trying to dismay me, but I don't get dismayed by a challenge.

"Great. I can do that."

"But stop as soon as you start doing it wrong," she added, "I don't want you to get into any bad habits."

At home, of course, I would conscientiously stop everything on the hour, go to the dining room table and take a swipe. I would do it wrong, with synergistic movement, not controlling isolated muscles. Stop. Back to my life. Repeat all day. Just another worthless frustration – as though I didn't have enough of that in my life. It was just that bad approach to therapy that resulted in this blog entry from about a year ago:

Failure

Posted September 2013

Stroke survivors are used to making lots of mistakes and doing nearly everything wrong or not at all (and doing nothing is also a failure).

Plus we go to therapy and are bombarded with instructions regarding how to fix everything we're doing wrong physically – walking mostly. And of course we can't do those correctly either.

And we also are in a very disappointing spot. We have gone from being bright, capable people to being bad at virtually everything; and getting it right is at some unknown point in the future, if ever.

Of course, our loved ones encourage us and praise our little improvements. But we are at a low (hopefully our all-time lowest) in our lives, and every time we pick ourselves up and try to do something again, we fail.

And, yes, survivors know all about success being not the number of times we fall, but the number of times we get back up. We learn that we must be our own best cheerleaders, but how does one cheer when the team is down 65-2, when every pass is an interception?

After a lifetime of excelling, I became suddenly incapable, incompetent, and appalled at my inadequacies. And I remain so.

Like my therapists, I constantly evaluate my implementation of the corrections my therapists have prescribed. Fail. I think constantly about what I'll try to fix the next time I walk. I try. Fail. I find out about a new therapy. I try it. Fail.

When my son, a linebacker, was in high school, he was captain of his football team. At the end of his senior year, he was awarded a regional Scholar-

Athlete award. His football coach had nominated him. At the awards ceremony, his coach sat at our table, and relayed to me why he had nominated Brian: At the start of every game throughout the season, he said, Brian would gather the team for a pep talk, always along the lines of "We can do this. Let's go out and get this done." Every time, his coach said, Brian acted as though his team was heading to the divisional Super Bowl, rather than being the 1-10 team they were at the end of the season. Brian had faith in his team and was completely convinced they could pull off the win every time.

That's how we survivors keep cheering despite a long history of failing: faith in ourselves.

It's when we lose that faith that we fail for the final time.

Yes, some therapists have been a complete waste of my time.

All along, I have done my own research and developed approaches/exercises that worked okay for me, except for the simple fact that my arm and hand are hardly more functional than my first day out of the rehab hospital. Even while I had a poor OT, I still had exercises and advice from previous ones – experienced ones. Throughout my recovery, I have cobbled together therapies and advice into what both makes sense to me *and* fits into my life. As I've said previously, it's a DIY approach to stroke rehab, and it's an approach every survivor must take, given that insurance companies stop paying for therapy after an arbitrary amount of time or when the survivor "plateaus." It's not clear yet how successful I'll be, but even if I'd toed the line the entire time and given up when multiple professionals said improvements were unlikely, I think it's unlikely I'd be any farther along than using my DIY technique. Obviously, there's no way of knowing. The final instruction I got from one OT is probably worth doing.

functional tasks for my left hand

Posted 25th October 2010

One of the things that my best OT said during my final OT session of the calendar year that stuck with me is: "Trying to use your left arm for day-to-day acts is what is going to bring it back."

On Sunday, after rowing in the gig [with Tom] with friends, I went home and used my left hand while I was shucking corn. Every week, Tom and I get vegetables from a local CSA farm and the delivery usually includes some ears of corn. In the past I have always left those for Tom to deal with because doing it one-handed didn't seem possible. Because Tom doesn't enjoy corn still on the cob, we always boil it, let it cool and then cut the kernals [kernels] off the cob. On Sunday, I decided to shuck it myself. I held the stalk end (which they had conveniently left about 4 to 6 inches long on each ear) in my left hand. I didn't grip it or anything as amazing as that, but I think my palm and gently grasping fingers provided enough friction that the ear stayed in place while I gently pulled the covering off leaf by leaf and tossed it in a paper bag. The silk ended up flying all over, but I did all eight myself and then put them in a pot of boiling water - Tom had put the full pot on the burner. I even broke off the 4 to 6 inches of stem by myself by using my right hand to hold the ear while I snapped the stalk off against my right thigh. When the timer went off after 5 minutes, I fished the ears out using tongs and left them on a plate to cool; previously, I would have put them in and promptly forgotten about them until the water spilled over and I could smell burning. And Tom got the vacuum cleaner for me and I cleaned up the silk (right-handed).

And Monday, I held a golf ball in my left hand for 5 minutes. It's not a functional act, but is something I could not do before.

Tuesday I carried two forks in my left hand from the kitchen to the library, where we were going to eat dinner, and today I carried a spoon when I wanted to have yogurt as a snack - I started by trying to carry the yogurt, but dropped it twice before settling on [carrying just] the spoon.

The current (summer 2014, 4.5 years post-stroke) status of my arm and hand is that I'm still using mirror therapy to try to open and close my hand; and in aquatic therapy, I'm learning to do the back crawl, which involves my entire arm, especially my shoulder and triceps. Once I can actually do the back crawl in my own non-standard way, along with opening and closing my hand, I think I'll be able to row a gig boat.

This is taking me years longer than I initially expected.

Intermission II: Pilgrimage

Posted 5th September 2010

Yesterday I started reading a book that a co-worker of Tom's loaned him - "A Leg to Stand On," by Oliver Sacks, a neurologist who also wrote, "The Man Who Mistook his Wife for a Hat," a collection of stories, which I have not read, about odd neurological patients he's had over the years. "A Leg to Stand On" is about his own recovery from an accident resulting from an encounter with a bull on a Norwegian mountainside. Alone, and with a destroyed knee that made his left leg useless, he remains analytical throughout his ordeal - calculating how fast he can travel on his butt using his arms to propel him down the mountainside, but predicting that he will make it back to civilization by nightfall or die from exposure. When he reaches a previously amusing sign saying, "Beware of bull," which he considers the halfway point, at twilight, he accepts that he will die, only to be spotted by a farmer and his son, and carried back to civilization, where he undergoes an operation to reconnect the tendons to his quadriceps. He is then hospitalized for two weeks, during which he realizes that he cannot control or feel his left leg at all, other than wiggling his toes; in fact, he ends up believing that his leg inside the cast is not there or is plaster or a combination of yucky decaying things, a belief that his surgeon considers rubbish and refuses to talk about. This "becoming a patient" for Dr. Sacks results in a soul-searching experience, which he calls a "pilgrimage," after a hospital official said to him, "Take it easy! The whole thing, going through it, is really a pilgrimage."

With a "pilgrimage" defined as "a journey to a sacred place," my experiences to return to myself, a state that feels like home, makes my former self sacred. At the time I had the stroke (I am still never tempted to call it "mine"), I knew that my life was blessed - not that God had singled me out to have nearly everything my heart desired, and more, but because I had nearly everything my heart desired, and more. I was filled with gratitude whenever I thought of my husband, kids, siblings, job, home life, health, friends, independence and circumstances, including the ability and time to row in Gloucester Harbor.

At that time, I went on a conditioning row (i.e., intense and requiring superb fitness, even for a rower) on a glorious day;

During our return from the Dogbar Breakwater at the mouth of the harbor, one of the other rowers complained when it was time for another set of power strokes. I don't remember what he said, but my response was: "If this isn't Heaven, I don't know what is."

That is the destination of my pilgrimage. That's all I want, but it is still far from reach...

Focusing on Leg Recovery

As I mentioned earlier, post-stroke, the recovery of the use of a leg is more likely than getting a hand/arm back. Not easy, but sooner and more likely, because of two factors: (1) bearing weight speeds recovery and (2) recovery requires repetition. Using a leg guarantees both of those. Also, one therapy goal before the release of a patient from the rehab hospital is usually for the patient to walk with an ankle-foot orthotic (AFO) and cane, but no other help. Re-entry into life is made easier that way.

I went home with an AFO, a monstrous plastic ankle and foot support that enabled me to stand and walk safely. It kept my ankle from rolling sideways and my toes from dragging on the floor. The monster also required that I wear shoes because I couldn't walk with the slick plastic directly on the floor.

One thing I didn't know about when I was fitted with an AFO in the rehab hospital, was that, as a long-term result, I would always wear an AFO. With my ankle held fixed at a right angle to prevent foot drop (dragging my toe), my peroneus muscles would atrophy and my soft tissue there would be destined to shorten and I would never be able to walk without a brace. I had no intention of wearing an AFO into the future, so, when I heard that, I immediately decided to ditch the thing ASAP.

One of the many problems associated with wearing my AFO was that it meant that when I woke up during the night in order to go to the bathroom, I needed to don all the paraphernalia – socks, AFO, and shoes – to get to the bathroom. To do that, I needed light and, at first, Tom's help. I felt awful, night after night, waking him in the early-morning hours so that I could go to the bathroom, especially given how many other tasks the stroke had burdened him with. Shouldn't he at least be able to sleep through the night?

Given that additional incentive, I worked toward being able to walk without the brace. Fundamentally, that work was practicing walking as much as I could, even with the AFO on: first inside the house, then outside. Inside, I had a track: ovals in our library, in the process of being renovated, circling the pile of two-by-fours in the center of the room.

While working on my walking, I asked my PT when I could attempt to go outside and walk a mile.

"Practice walking to the end of your driveway and back," she responded. "How pathetically short," I thought.

By April 2012 (2.5 years post-stroke), I was up to walking 2 miles – usually with a friend. What it took, really, was persistence and time – things every stroke survivor has.

The next step was ditching the AFO and rewiring my brain to connect to and strengthen my peroneus muscles:

peroneus (longus and brevus) muscles

We have two muscles at 11 o'clock on our calf (in the front of the left shin; 2 o'clock on our right shin) - the peroneus longus and peroneus brevus - which pull up the toes on the outside of our feet. Until I can control and strengthen those on my left leg, I must wear my brace and use my cane; otherwise, my toes will drop and drag and my ankle will buckle.

… To control and strengthen them [my peroneus muscles], I do myriad exercises every day:

112

1. bridges that include rotating my hips, as in the hula.

2. lying down flat, pulling my toes toward my nose [flexing my foot]; lifting my toes evenly with my knee bent at a right angle; repeating again with my knee halfway between flat and a right angle.

3. leaning against a wall and doing not-so-deep knee bends (that's for my quads, too).

4. attaching my electronic stimulator and letting that contract the muscles, on and off for 20 minutes.

5. sitting, lifting my knee without my foot swinging out.

Plus, when I use the rowing machine, I try to keep my left knee from banging into my right, staying about 4 inches away. Also, as I walk and go down stairs, I work on keeping my toe pointing straight forward when its tendency is to point in [spasticity at work]. And here's an exercise I made up for myself: Every evening, I stand brace-less, behind a heavy, upholstered high-backed chair, stabilizing myself with my right arm on the chair-back, and try to raise myself onto the toes of both my feet. That simulates how my foot should move as I walk, so I figured it would be helpful.

Another technique I find helpful when trying to isolate the muscle I should be working on, is to perform the task with my strong, perfect leg or arm and shoot for the comparable muscle in my weak side ...

After becoming confident in my ability to walk AFO-less, I started always walking brace-less, but with a cane, inside our house. Once I was able to do that easily, I decided to tackle the stairs. Down was the challenge, which I first did down a few steps leading to the back door. Next was a full staircase, made as safe as I possibly could.

A whole flight of stairs without the brace

Posted 2nd March 2011

Yesterday I tackled going down our back stairs without my brace. I chose that staircase because it is carpeted, and I wore rubber-soled slippers so that I was less likely to slip. Although I had no one hovering to spot me, there were two people in the house in case I had any trouble ...

After I could go up and down stairs, I tried for the next obvious step:

walking outside without the brace

Posted 15th March 2011

Today, in addition to walking around my house (including up and down the stairs a half dozen times) without my brace, my friend Pat, my dog, Turbo, and I walked to the end of my street and back, which is about a half-mile, without it. I know that I don't walk properly ... so I concentrated on lifting my knee and stepping heel-toe. Again, like much of what I do, it wasn't pretty, but it felt like an accomplishment, something that can often be in short supply. And I was tired at the end, but nothing that tea and a brownie couldn't fix. Then Pat and I worked on organizing the books in the new library and, to carry books, I had to go without my cane, which was not as scary as it was last Thursday when my PT told my OT that I didn't need it and made me leave it in the PT room.

Last year at this time, I both ventured out by myself for the first time AND, on a different day, walked to the

> end of my road and back for the first time [in my AFO last year, but brace-less this year]. Progress!!!

I went without a brace for nearly a year. Unlike other stroke survivors with hemiparesis, keeping my ankle stable, not foot drop, was the most unnerving problem I had. I worried with each trip I made down stairs anywhere, and I had trouble with my ankle on uneven surfaces – lawns, beaches, loose gravel, and cobbled paths.

The next time I saw my physiatrist and explained the situation, he recommended finding a smaller, lighter carbon-fiber AFO, and he wrote an order for PT to evaluate braces, get a new one, and have follow-up PT. I went to a local clinic and found the best PT of all time. She lined up a brace specialist to come talk to us. I had one objection or other to every brace sample he had. Smaller standard AFO's and the carbon-fiber ones both kept my ankle locked in position, which meant I'd lose my ability to walk without it. One jabbed into the back of my knee. Both of those issues were problems with the AFO I already had and hated about it. We talked with him about electronic braces – I had used one type in previous PT sessions and knew I didn't like that product. Another, though – the Bioness L300 – was appealing. The brace rep brought a left-side sample on his next visit, and I tried it. It immediately stimulated my peroneus muscles, everting (pointing out) my foot, stabilizing my ankle, and keeping my toes up. I fell in love. Of course, it was expensive, and my insurance didn't cover it, even though it could very well stimulate my peroneus muscles so that I would one day walk safely without any aid.

But Bioness has a rent-to-own program, so I signed up.

115

I ended up purchasing a unit. Once I was using it, the ability to walk safely – even on uneven surfaces - seemed worth the cost.

I still use this brace now all of the time, including walking around my house with it, but without a cane, unless I'm going up or down stairs. I no longer have a PT, and have no idea how to prepare myself to go up or down steps with my L300, but without a cane. When I asked other stroke survivors how to deal with stairs without a cane, they all had the same suggestion: use a railing, and descend backwards if the railing is on the wrong side.

What I really am asking is how to go up and down stairs with my Bioness, but no other aid. To me, using a railing is just like using a cane. What I want is to be able to handle two steps up into a building without a railing (Massachusetts building code requires a flight of three or more steps to have a railing). And to handle curbs when I'm out – up one step, down one step. Given no PT to help me work on it, this is going to be another DIY project.

Four years post-stroke, and that's my current leg/walking goal. Yes, recovery requires all – and maybe more – of the patience you can muster.

To row, though, I need no more improvement in my leg. Since being released from rehab, I have been able to, both with and without an AFO or the L300, walk down the hill to the rowing pier, go down the gangway to the floating dock without help from anyone. Then, with help steadying both me and the boat, I can climb in and move carefully to my seat. During the row, I'm able to keep both feet on the footrest and push on it. Upon returning to the dock at the end of the row, I can, again, with some steadying, climb out and walk to my car. Further improvement in my leg would facilitate climbing into and around on the boat, but is not required.

Throughout this ordeal, I have tried to identify and appreciate small steps (no pun intended). Improvements, though hardly noticeable sometimes, keep my hope alive – that improvements happen and are hardly noticed; in nearly 5 years, I have progressed from not being able to walk the morning I had the stroke, to being capable of going freely out into the world. Yes, it's with a brace and cane, but to me that's better than nothing. Again, I want to get the task done, regardless of how I do it.

Sometimes the steps in my leg recovery are huge. For Saebo therapy, I was able to travel by train to and from Boston every week, which required all the stamina and courage I had. I was also able to travel to Sweden with my family, without a brace, and I flew alone to Florida to visit a friend.

And sometimes the steps are hardly noticeable, as they were after a year of using the Bioness leg brace:

unnoticed progress

Posted 21 August 2013

At my last OT session, I was tapping my left foot while I waited for my OT to pull over a mirror; well, I was pulling my toes up in a rhythmic fashion anyway. My OT asked why I was wearing a Bioness L300 if I could do that. I didn't have a good answer. Then, when I went to my physiatrist for my Botox evaluation, I talked to him about it. He watched me walk both with and without the L300 turned on. His conclusion was that, although not perfect, the device has been doing its job and training my peroneus muscles to work almost properly. Now it's still worth wearing because it helps my stability, especially going down stairs, but that should develop, too. And I have noticed lately that I can do braceless what I was not able to do before: walk on wet, packed sand and on lawn; very carefully. So, I agree that it has been doing its job, without me even noticing.

As you have seen, my experiences have been a roller coaster ride – both emotionally and physically. It is inevitable when tackling a difficult challenge. I try, though, to focus on the step forward, not the two steps back. In stroke recovery, I have accepted that I will fail. A lot. What happens after a failure is a reflection of persistence: after I fall, I stand up and try again.

As I've explained before, falling/failure has been my constant companion, but it hasn't stopped me yet. And not all of recovery has been an ordeal.

Recovering fun

Survivors lose more than the ability to use a hand/arm, to walk, do their jobs well, drive, clean house, do home maintenance, and the other obvious results of losing control of half-a-body. We also lose our abilities to do many activities that bring us joy: our hobbies and recreation. Some are athletic pursuits, like rowing, running, dancing, golfing, bike riding, swimming, and rock climbing. Others are activities that have become too logistically difficult, like painting en plein air, blueberry picking, walking the dog, and traveling. And then there are the things that are possible in theory, but more challenging one-handed than people think: gardening and cooking.

Stroke recovery guru Peter Levine says that survivors who have specific goals about activities they love will make more progress than those who work on capabilities that don't apply to favorite pastimes. Here's a reiteration:

17th November 2010 [one year post-stroke]

I got back on the horse [after falling off the rowing machine when I was in a hurry the previous day] and went 3 miles on the rowing machine this morning - in 42:07, which I think is 14:24 per mile. Next time I will go 4 miles, then 5. My goal is 5.5 miles in less than 5.5 times my 5-mile rate. Instead of being in a hurry today, I woke up at 5:15 and started rowing just before 6.

Yesterday I finished Peter Levine's Stronger After Stroke, a book about stroke recovery from the point of view of a stroke rehab specialist... I'm very glad I read it because ... it contains a comprehensive overview of our choices and treatment options plus encourages survivors to take charge of and responsibility for their own recovery. It has a chapter on motivation that includes the idea that someone who was out-of-shape and unconcerned about his/her fitness before the stroke can hardly be expected to muster the motivation to work hard to get to a never-before-experienced fitness level. On the other hand, athletes know how to work hard to reach a fitness goal, so they can be expected to do the same after a stroke.

He also ties motivation and recovery to a survivor's passion - someone who was passionate about golf before the stroke can expect better recovery as he/she works toward the ability to return to playing golf. I see that that is true for me ... rowing is the driving force during my recovery process.

According to Levine, incremental improvements that are barely noticeable day by day yield successful results as long as the improvement contributes to once again doing something that is meaningful to the survivor. In my own life, this translates into focusing my work on my grip and release so that every day I should push the limits of what I can already do, with the short-term [overly optimistic to call it a "short-term" goal, it turned out, given that I still cannot do it 4 years later] goal of grasping a PVC pipe that is the same circumference as an oar. He also stresses that endless repetitive acts are required to allow recovery. I have decided to keep my pipe with me all day long at home so that I can grip it as often as possible.

By mid-July 2011 (1.5 years post-stroke), I was able to get back to some tasks in one of my favorite pastimes - gardening:

avocation and vocation

I spent yesterday gardening - I'll admit mostly weeding - in glorious weather. Because I could. It was the first full day of gardening post-stroke. I never did spend a day gardening last summer because it was too difficult to stay close enough to the ground. Last summer's gardening consisted of either (1) bending at the waist and reaching with my unaffected hand, which tired out my unaffected leg faster than I thought it would (I admire my unaffected leg because it is incredibly strong, and patient too) or (2) sitting on a small rolling stool my husband bought me. The stool's limitation is that, even with its wheels, it's hard to move it around the garden; I cannot roll it while sitting on it because my AFO digs into the back of my bent knee and I end up more inclined to push myself off the stool rather than moving the stool. So I end up standing and pulling the cart to a new spot and sitting again. That's a LOT of deep-knee bends, which are easier for me this summer than last.

Are my current weeds the result of an ignored garden last summer? I think so. So this year, it is even more important to keep up. When we bought this house 6 years ago, it had spent the past maybe 40 years getting to its overgrown state, and we spent years carving out garden from the jungle. We had made significant progress; and it was quite lovely the summer before I had the stroke. Not anymore.

The summer after the stroke, some of my siblings came one weekend and weeded, then spread mulch - 7 yards - over the newly weeded beds and paths, so the garden was acceptable until crabgrass and a few other nasties sprouted in mid-summer. The good news re using the "ignore" gardening method is that I did not deadhead, and plants like dianthus went to seed and serendipitously spread to perfect places among the rocks, including down below an outcropping above a path.

Yesterday, I carried/tossed a cushion (the atrophied gluteus muscles on my affected side have not yet bulked up, which leaves me with little padding on my left cheek and discourages rock-sitting) around the garden so that I could sit on it on rocks and weed around that rock. Again, lots of deep-knee bends, but I did them just fine, using my cane to keep myself from pitching forward as I stood. In a particularly wide patch of crabgrass, I set up a low beach chair - again, my carrying method was heaving the closed chair, then following it to its landing place and repeating the process. I "carried" the tools, including a couple of sharp ones by shutting them inside the folded chair before tossing the chair. I am afraid of tripping and falling onto one tool in particular - It's a Japanese hand hoe: a long-handled one with a bent blade that is blunt, but has a pointed end at a right angle to the handle. Falling on it, my weight would negate the bluntness of the blade, I'm sure. So I toss it instead of carrying.

Tossing is often my preferred "carrying" method, even indoors. I drop soft objects - dirty laundry, dog toys and jackets - down the center well of the front staircase, where they land on the first landing (perfect name, right?)

My very first OT called my problem-solving approach "inventive," something I am proud of - I particularly enjoy when an OT tells me that I "should have been" an OT - I think it's high praise. Part of me DOES want to be an OT or PT after this ordeal is over. There was a nurse in rehab who'd had a stroke 6 years before, which made me want to be a nurse in a rehab facility. When that [yearning] happens, I have to remind myself that I am a writer - that's my true identity, pre-stroke and post-stroke. This stroke will not derail me from that - it will contribute to it.

While one might consider writing a hobby for me, it is not – writing is my vocation, although I do have it as a hobby as I write my blog; reading, though, is one of my most important hobbies.

Just after the stroke, although I had no identifiable language deficits, I did have trouble reading – my eyes fell off the right end of one printed line and I couldn't tell where to pick up the line at the left margin; the solution I devised was to hold a bookmark sideways under the line I was reading, then drop it down one line as I went. I did it on my laptop monitor too, while I read email.

There was another reading issue: being able to hold onto/control the book, especially while turning pages. Reading a paperback, I would keep the back of the spine against my middle finger, with my other fingers inside the book, holding it open. Hardcovers were out of the question, unless they were very thin.

Then, to turn a page, my thumb, on the right-hand facing page, would have to pull that page to the left while my ring finger and pinky caught the page under them. That's the moment that, inevitably, I would drop the book. After swearing and picking the book up again, it would take me sometimes approaching an hour to find my place to continue reading. I generally used that as a time to stop, knowing that the next time I wanted to read it, I'd be searching all over again, but procrastinating the hassle. I tried using a bookmark placed beyond where I was in the book to indicate that I was somewhere preceding that, but of course the bookmark fluttered out as the book fell to the floor, so that didn't solve anything.

The final, and successful, solution was to buy an iPad. It works wonderfully for me except for reading in bed. I still haven't found a position I can lie in and keep the book in view. Sitting up with my back to the headboard seems to be a good solution except I can't move my rear end up that far toward the head of the bed. Atrophied glutes on my left side keep me from being able to wiggle my hips and butt-walk backwards. Ditto using a triangular back-rest pillow. But reading on the iPad is far better than the real book. The perfect solution would be to project the text from the iPad to the ceiling so that I could read it while flat on my back.

Another of my favorite recreational activities is to visit college friends at their cottage on a small lake in New Hampshire, which we generally do a couple times each summer. The stroke nixed a few traditions for me there, including sleeping in the tree-house, because of its ladder access, kayaking, swimming and lolling in the sun on the floating raft. Horseshoes, though, was still possible in early July 2010:

Horseshoes

It being the Fourth of July weekend, Tom, Turbo and I headed to the cabin on a NH lake of friends of ours for Friday and Saturday ... I walked into deeper and deeper water. My original intention was to wade in far enough to test whether I can tread water, but as I walked, the water became colder and the idea of treading water less appealing; ... and I headed back to shore ...

One of the most endearing attributes of the Churchills' cottage is the horseshoe set-up in sand next to the cabin. Before my venture into the water, we played horseshoes - Judie and I against Tom and John. Horseshoes appealed to me precisely because it seemed to require a challenging combination of balance and coordination that perhaps I didn't have. The shoes are seriously heavy and I had to heave each with all my might while visually focusing on the distant pin (although John made the women's distance half that of the men's) after rocking front to back to line up the throw and stepping/standing without my cane (because the horseshoe was in my right hand) - it had the potential to make me lose my balance, so I was eager to try. And I did not lose my balance even once! We lost, though, 21-18. Which means Judie and I did all right. The biggest challenge turned out to be keeping Turbo out of harm's way - he somehow managed to nearly always be in the line of fire ...

Another pastime to recover is enjoying romance.

Nearly 40 years ago, I was blessed to find the man I have been married to for 32 years. He has been my caregiver throughout this ordeal - this sudden, and painful, deflection of our life plan. From the beginning, he has exhibited all the wonderful characteristics one hopes for in a spouse during hard times. And some. Spending time with him is one of my favorite pastimes. Three months post-stroke was February:

Valentine's Day

Posted 14th February 2010

Neither Tom nor I have ever been romantic. In our nearly 28 years of marriage, we've given each other a handful of valentines (combined) and our most fun [wedding] anniversary involved walking to a local restaurant for dinner, the two of us and both kids, all together to celebrate.

Today [Valentine's Day three months post-stroke], though, I wanted to walk out in the garden, and Tom humored me. ... We have a granite outcropping off the south side of the house, with a path winding down to

125

the lower levels, including a level area with a white-painted metal-and-glass table and chairs. That was my destination. We went out the back door, then over the rough terrain to the granite ledge. The endeavor was a challenge ... because my quad cane (with its four feet) was not stable on the uneven ground and because my right leg tired from bearing most of my weight most of the time. About halfway down, Tom went to fetch one of the chairs for me to rest on. He set it down in the sun along the path and put his down vest on it to insulate me from the cold metal. As I sat there, he leaned against the arm of the chair and I threw my right arm around his legs, and we enjoyed the warmth of the sun and our contact. Once rested, we continued down the path to the lower level and I made my way to another chair there. Again, Tom cushioned the seat for me with his vest. Standing there in the sun, protected from the breeze by the surrounding rocks, was not quite warm enough for him, though, so he headed back to the house for a jacket, returning with chocolates and a glass of red wine to share. He pulled up another chair next to mine and we sat, enjoying the pretty [pinkish granite] rocks, view of the ocean, sunshine, bittersweet chocolate, sips of wine, and companionship, and talking about which locust trees and wild roses should stay and which should go, based on his desire to clear paths amid a cluster of rocks standing like statues just below the level area.

Socializing is also a fun way to spend our recovery time. After I had the stroke, friends and family - and even some strangers - rallied around me and helped encourage and inspire me, as well as helping out with the overwhelming tasks Tom and I confronted going home: cooking, housekeeping, getting to appointments, etc. In particular, I especially enjoyed being with friends while they were *not* helping me out — the ones who invited me to go out to lunch or dinner, or to play mah jongg or Bananagrams, or invited themselves over to talk and/or walk our dogs. One particular outing stands out:

Girls just want to have fun!

Last Friday, I went with three girlfriends to a "Mama Gena" show in Springfield. Mama Gena is a persona created by Regena Thomashauer, founder of "The School of Womanly Arts," which teaches women to adore themselves and all other women. Bottom-line: Mama Gena considers every woman a sister and every woman a goddess. Self-introductions MUST be along the lines of "I'm Sister Goddess Barbara," etc.

This is not a mode of thought I was interested in pre-stroke. While I appreciated being cheerful, energetic, active and athletic – components required in order to be attractive – I was not interested in over-the-top femininity or sensuality.

Post-stroke, though, I find myself missing admiring looks, and spend most of the time feeling inadequate, as women go.

My saint of a husband does not help at times like that; he despises dealing with me when I'm obsessing about shoes or dresses or how this pair of jeans looks compared to that. His attitude is that I've had a stroke and that dressing up is a waste because I will always end up looking like I had a stroke. True, but it makes me sad.

But I have a very girly girlfriend who arranged the outing to see Mama Gena. A few days beforehand, I asked her what I should wear. "Pink," she replied instantly. Now, pink is not a color in my wardrobe – black, I've got, everything you could ever want in black. For color I've got every shade of blue and green, plus a few red items. Pink? No pink. The closest to pink I have is a BLACK dress with RED roses and a RUFFLE at the bottom.

When I went to her house to get dressed, I took that black dress, a little black cardigan and a black cape (think: 1950s nurse); of course, there were also my black walking shoes and socks. For starters, it took me 15 minutes and a lot of tears [crying, not rips] to get the clothing into a bag to take to Lisa's house; I HATED those frigging wadded clothes by the time I left my house, But when I got to Lisa's, she had a gauzy electric blue dress that was too big for her despite the fact it was a Small ...It fit me perfectly – long-sleeved and buttoned up the front. Did I mention it was gauzy? Gauzy, as in see-through. "What do you think of it being see-through?" I asked. Her response? "See-through with those black panties and a hot-pink bra? PERFECT for Mama Gena!" Obviously, I lied about the pink issue – I do have a hot-pink pullover bra, but it doesn't usually fall into the category of "pink clothes" when I'm picking out an outfit.

Given the brilliant blue of the dress and its fabulous fit, I decided I was presentable, but just in case, threw on [actually, I labored to get it on, then work the brass the brass closures of my black cape. We then picked up two other friends – one a gorgeous and sexy Brazilian and the other a pretty and slender woman who always looks well put-together [Both dressed in pink, with ruffles].

As we got out of the car in Springfield, Lisa handed around pink feather boas that we all wrapped around our necks. Each of them tweaked mine to improve it.

At the start of the show, Mama Gena, [dressed in a tiny pink sequined dress] was carried in by half a dozen shirt-less buff guys, with "Girls Just Want to Have Fun" [Cindy Lauper] as the music. The show, which was interactive, was also raunchy, funny and, yet, it somehow built our self-esteem. With 100 women watching, we got to talk about our desires, how to tell a desire from a goal, learned how to brag and how to put together a "pleasure basket" for our bedside. Women talked about pleasure and feeling luscious, about being single and having sex (which Mama called "research"), about being married and having sex. She had us all stand, point to our butts and say, "I have a hot ass." "Smoking" was also an acceptable adjective. And we laughed and laughed, increasing our nitric acid level, she said, something laughing has in common with orgasm. At least in women; she didn't mention men, not in that context. Maybe it's why women fall in love with men who make them laugh.

Recovering rowing

In my quest to recover the ability to have fun, rowing has been number-one on my list.

While rowing a pilot gig boat was likely the cause of my artery dissection, which led to having a stroke, it is still an important goal of mine to return to rowing – as a regular, strong member of a crew. There are particular rows I want to do: early-morning conditioning, to Ten-Pound Island for a picnic (or wine and cheese), moonlight, and novice training (to help out), among others. To do that, I must be able to competently row on my own (i.e., without Tom). Having some help, getting in and out of the gig, for example, would be acceptable, along with not being able to haul the boat to the dock to be secured so that other rowers can disembark. I accept that I will never be captain or cox; I think neither I nor any other rower would likely be comfortable with that.

Being "stroke," that is, the rower who sets the pace for the others, though, is particularly attractive to me – because of semantics, I think. It requires that the rower establish a strong, rhythmic stroke to be followed by the other rowers and at the pace specified by the cox. It's a challenge because the rower stroking is expected to be precise every stroke of the entire row; it is an hour of sustained scrutiny. Before having a stroke, I had acted as stroke for 20 minutes on only one single row (the cox decided three of us would practice being stroke); I was stressed the entire time, but did fine.

From the beginning of my recovery, I have focused on the skills required to be back in the boat without one-on-one help.

The first goal I had was to have the strength and stamina to row for an hour, the length of a standard row. An old college friend who lives in New Hampshire came to visit one day with a Concept II rowing machine in a pickup; he and his wife set it up and I tried it out for 10 minutes, with the help of an Ace bandage holding my hand on the handle.

With the help of my OT, we devised a schedule that took me from 5 minutes of rowing per day for a week, adding 5 minutes per session each week until I hit 60 minutes a day. She wanted me to start very unambitiously and gradually increase, while on my own I probably would have started trying for an hour.

During the first week of the rowing schedule, I made this entry …

rowing machine

Posted 11th August 2010

This morning, I went about 30 minutes without my leg brace while getting up, having coffee and getting dressed. I also went without it going down the stairs (a first!), although I chose the safer stairway and Tom went back to hovering in front of me as I descended. … And I used the rowing machine for 15 minutes, also without my leg brace. Through it all, my ankle stayed strong and straight, without buckling and rolling as it used to at every single step.

That's the second day so far this week that I've rowed 15 minutes on the machine. The biggest challenge in the procedure is keeping my left hand attached to the handle.

As my ability to row longer on the machine progressed, there was concomitant progress on other fronts -

specifically walking without my brace, which has been a long-standing goal, but not one needed to row. This entry shows a bit about how those two goals are/were intertwined in time, plus a bit about the deterioration of my status at work ...

60-minute rows

Posted 13th October 2010

I'm in the midst of my first week doing 60 minutes of rowing on the rowing machine and today was my second day accomplishing that. It was nice that this accomplishment coincided with the 11-month mark following the stroke, which was yesterday, because it seems to me that it means I've made a lot of progress on my pilgrimage since that life-changing day.

Also, last week I resigned my position as general manager at the newspaper - an action that was heartbreaking for me and difficult for my boss also (he regrets the loss of the way things used to be, which I just haven't been able to manage to get back to since the stroke, despite my best efforts). I will remain working at the paper, though, because I proposed going back to copy editor and my boss agreed... the change makes me happy, although it often makes me cry, too.

As Tom often says, I've lost an awful lot and it's no wonder that I'm upset whenever another loss gets added to the list. So although I've lost the favorite job I've ever had, at the same time, I've managed to build my strength and stamina enough to row 60 minutes at a time.

Although my goal is to row in the gig, which will be an enormous accomplishment, also rewarding was *seeing* the gig for the first time post-stroke. I posted this about 6 months after the stroke ...

Gloucester Gig Rowers

Posted 29th May 2010

Tom took me over to the Gloucester Maritime Heritage Center, where the club's boats are moored, so that I could attend a new-rower orientation class as an observer. There was a lot of activity since, in addition to the orientation, the new teen rowing class was being held, some repair work was being done on the boat trailer and the foot rests of the second boat were being varnished. Going there [to the center] brought tears to my eyes, as did seeing rowers I had seen little of all winter.

Some of the rowers I see regularly - some are friends who visit frequently and drive me to therapy and other places I need to go; some are on the Steering Committee with me, so we see each other there monthly; the others I've rowed with and raced with and socialized with at events. All of them were a pleasure to see again.

That was *seeing* the gig, but then there was *being in* the gig. I posted this at the end of May ...

first time back in the gig

Posted 30th May 2010

Not only was today's 9 a.m. row my first time back in the Siren Song, it was my first ride as a passenger ...

This morning, Tom and Turbo dropped me off, Tom helped me zip and latch my PFD, and I headed to the boat to be a passenger. A few rowers helped me as I made my way down the gangway to the float where the Siren Song is moored. The SS was just returning from an 8 a.m. row, and two of the male rowers stayed to help me climb on board. With a few people stabilizing the boat and keeping it close to the dock, I sat on the gunwale adjacent to my seat and swung my legs in, feet onto the floorboards, which were not askew; Stephen straightened out the floorboards for me and cleared a bumper and water bottle from the space at my feet.

... Being a passenger gave me a unique perspective: a rower in any seat faces the stern to row, but as a passenger, I faced the bow, with all the rowers and the coxswain behind me. In a pilot gig like our club's, the seats are numbered 1 through 6 from the bow. Seat 6 is just forward of the cox, who sits at the stern to man the rudder, which [steers] the boat. The oars for seats 6, 4 and 2 stick out the starboard side of the boat, while the odd-numbered ones are out on the port side ...

To be out on the still, slightly rippled water this morning, smelling the salt air up close, with just the rumble of passing boats and the creak and thud of the oars moving between the thole pins (which act as oarlocks) was close to heaven. Being one rower short (plus me as extra weight) made the row more of a workout for the rowers, but they ... quickly [made] it out of the Inner Harbor to the Greasy Pole. The remaining row was around Ten-Pound Island, where we took a rest on the far side, and back to the dock. We spent the rest period laughing ... Despite the laughter, I started to get chilled at that point and was happy when the cox started the rowers toward home.

Sitting in the bow, listening to the oars all in synch, made me miss rowing all over again - I miss pulling on

134

the oar, working up a sweat, feeling the blade pull through the water and propel the boat forward, my whole body working in unison with the rest of the crew - that's what I miss. And that hole is not filled by rowing with strangers in the adaptive rowing program [which I tried and had a negative experience with] or going as a passenger in the Siren Song.

While docking, I kept being tempted to help - to grab the dock as we approached and the two rowers closest to the bow came forward and stepped to the dock to pull the boat in; if we had been docking on my right side instead of my left, I definitely would have grabbed it, but the dock was on my left side, so there wasn't much I could do.

Climbing out of the boat at the end was somehow easier than climbing in. Again, I sat on the gunwale and swung my legs, this time from the boat to the dock. At one point, I felt myself falling onto my left side on the dock. "I'm falling to my left," I said. Bill, standing on the dock behind me, reached for me and got me under my arms. "No, you're not," he said, as he hoisted me to my feet. My legs were shaking under me (as they do when they are fatigued) as he handed me my cane and I headed up the gangway. At the top of the gangway is the most challenging step: a variable-sized step up to the main platform of the pier. The gangway runs from the pier down to the floating dock where the boats are tied, so the size of the step at the top and the angle of the ramp are both dependent on the tide. Today, I'd say the step was about 12 inches, but I made it up okay.

By September, I was ready to venture out using a splint my OT had made me to loosely attach my hand to the oar so that I could row – or act as though I was rowing, at least. I hand-selected my crew and scheduled my first "real" row ...

135

my first row

Posted 26th September 2010

Any success I experienced today was entirely due to the Gloucester Gig Rowers, my OT and my husband. I went rowing this morning at 10 - the weather could not have been better: warm, sunny, no wind - it was lovely. Bart and Tom helped me get into the gig. Chip was cox and Esther sat in the seat behind me - 1 - while Tom sat in 3, facing me. As instructed by my OT, once we were out in the harbor, ready to row, with my hook splint strapped on my arm, I went through the motions for the first minute out of the water, making sure I could use the hook to move the oar without having the resistance of the water. The way it actually worked was that, as usual, my right arm took over and did most of the work, while nearly every time I pulled with my left arm, the hook slid off the oar. In addition, my fingers were smashed between the splint, the oar and Tom's hand over mine; my thumb, especially, was uncomfortably positioned between the splint and the oar.

At the beginning of the row, I explained that, using my rowing machine, I typically row 22 strokes a minute, although after a warm-up period, I shoot for a [typical] pace of 28, but rarely get there. The cox and the stroke (Clem, who is like a human metronome when he's setting the pace) agreed that we'd try to go about 20 or 22 strokes per minute, which sounded perfect to me.

After about 10 minutes of rowing across calm water, I asked for a break because I was worried I was blistering/abrading the fingers on my left hand. During the break, Tom, Esther and I tried to get a rowing glove on my uncooperative left hand, then, when I couldn't straighten my fingers enough to go through the holes in the glove, settled on sandwiching the glove between the splint and my hand as cushioning.

At the end of the break, I said it was time to head back, which surprised some of the rowers because I usually have such a can-do attitude. I, though I was very pleased to be out rowing, knew that I could not have done it at all without Tom, who stood and set my oar on command, repositioned my hand and hook back onto the oar every minute or so, handed me his handkerchief when I needed it, and so on. As grateful as I was to have him there to help me, I would have preferred to be self-sufficient. So, knowing that, as is, I am not capable of rowing on my own, I thought it was time to end the experiment and go back to the dock.

Once we were back, Chip opened a bottle of champagne and toasted me and my persistence, along with Tom for being a "stand-up guy," which I thought was very sweet ... Although many people acknowledge the work Tom does looking out for me and I often express my gratitude to him for the sacrifices he makes for me, it was heartwarming to have someone else verbalize it in front of him and others.

I know that he appreciated the toast for its sincerity and the acknowledgement of his supportive nature.

But it was momentous: going out rowing in a pilot gig for the first time following a stroke. When I climbed out and was standing on the dock with both Bart and Tom holding onto me, I started to sob, hardly able to believe that I had accomplished such a thing.

Periodically through the following three seasons (2011, 2012 and 2013), I went out with a small group of friends for perhaps a total of 5 rows per season. In the meantime, Tom has worked on designing a splint that helps hold my hand to the oar. The trick is to create something that allows me to pull the oar toward me, but also allows for a quick release if I/my oar get in trouble. The goal is to let me both pull on the oar without coming off *and* pull on the oar in order to come off; in effect, hanging on tight when I want to and letting go when I want to. The problem with being firmly attached is that if my oar crabs or somehow goes awry, my shoulder might be dislocated and/or I could end up in the water.

In the 2013 rowing season, after several attempts with alternate splints, we returned to the technique of Tom holding my hand onto the oar – attempting to keep my fingers open and wrapped around the oar; we will also use that technique as the 2014 season gets underway. With my fingers unfurling and getting squashed between the oar and Tom's grip, it's not anything like a permanent solution. Although it does not meet my goal of rowing independently, it's the best I can do now with my fingers not straightening to open my hand. Holding onto the oar by myself is the permanent solution.

Will I ever get there?

Intermission III: The "New Normal"

Along this journey, several people (most recently, my OT) have referred to coping with post-stroke life as establishing a "new normal" so that a survivor can move forward. To me, that sounds as though I just have to get used to it. Simple, right?

When we were 42, my best friend from college died after a prolonged struggle with breast cancer. She had spent several years in a pretty bad way, including living with the results of a metastasis to her brain. As hard as she fought and as determined as she was to beat it (the youngest of her three children was 6 when she died, the most compelling incentive ever), for a long time it was clear to me that the end was approaching. When she died, though, I had trouble incorporating her absence into my reality. I would wake up in the morning having forgotten that she had died; after a little while, I would remember. That went on for weeks until finally one morning, it didn't have to come to me, I just knew it from the start.

Having a stroke was similar – while I was in the rehab hospital, I would wake up in the morning and have to remember that I couldn't move my left side. It happened in my dreams, too – for a long time after the stroke, I didn't dream at all, but then after a few months or so, I started to. At first, I wasn't disabled in my dreams. I liked that because I understood it to mean that I had not incorporated being disabled into my definition of myself.

I don't remember how long that lasted, but I do remember the first dream in which I was disabled: Turbo was still small and I had been anxious about him being a starter in a coyote's dinner. In my dream, I went outside with Turbo, and once he got to the grass, a coyote rushed him and pounced. Fortunately, I had my cane with me, so I started toward the coyote with my cane in the air (and happy to have it), ready to whack him/her, but couldn't proceed – I had a cane, so I must have been disabled, and, given that, I couldn't get to, much less attack, the coyote, there was nothing I could do to stop him/her. Or, in a dream-like fashion, did I manage to get there and break them up after all? At the time, I'm sure I remembered what happened in the dream, but I don't remember right now. In dreams since then – and now - I am disabled.

That's what I think people mean when they refer to a "new normal" – defining life in a whole new way, or even defining myself in a new way – waking up in the morning having already incorporated a new life/self in my psyche.

I think of the stroke as causing a reset in my life, a tap on the arc of my path so that my trajectory changed. While I haven't done a 180-degree turn, I also have not simply taken giant steps backward. Of course, on my previous path there was no likelihood that I was going to reach my final intended destination (best-selling author) anyway. After all, I was certainly not living my life with the precision of a missile launch – it was messy, with poorly fleshed-out parts and poorly implemented bits.

In my life, though, this stroke was a disturbance that set me back on the track to being a writer, ultimately the correct destination for me. Despite my original life's intention of having a career as a writer, my pre-stroke professional path as a manager was not going to take me there, and I had been unlikely to leave that path for the correct one, not inclined to jump from the safety of the newspaper to a writer's life. The stroke made being a writer possible.

Yes, unlike my early post-stroke contention that this stroke SHOULD NOT HAVE struck me, today I can actually put on some distorted glasses that allow me to see one result of the stroke – the heartbreaking loss of my job - as a blessing.

But, one question in my life will always be: Are the benefits that came from the stroke worth the concomitant losses?

All along, I have called this ordeal a "nightmare," but it hasn't been. Don't get me wrong: It certainly hasn't been a "dream" in the positive definition of the word. "Alternate universe" and "parallel path" are better (and non-judgmental) descriptions. My stroke experience has been a story, a saga that I never expected to tell.

My new normal is – as was my old one – me enthusiastically doing the best I can with what I have been given in my current situation. Certainly what I've been given, what my best is, and my current situation have all changed, but I – that internal nugget of "Barb" - is still there – the scrappy, opinionated (and even smart) liberal New Englander who can get lost even when driving straight.

That combination of factors has created my new normal, my new life. And it's a good one.

Emotional recovery

Post-stroke, looking ahead toward the unknown is daunting. Looking back, we focus on our losses. Living here and now is a combination of the two, mixed with disappointment.

In January 2009 (2 months post-stroke), between laughs, a visiting, and relatively new, friend shook her head and peered into my eyes.

"Are you always like this?" she asked.

If I'd wanted praise and a pat on the back, I could have disingenuously questioned what she meant, and she would have spoken admiringly about my attitude, but I knew what she meant: both of us were relaxed, light-hearted and enjoying ourselves.

Instead I said, "It's not so bad."

Like lots of other stroke survivors, I have tried to cope well, even though our new lives are challenging and full of frustrations. One of my challenges has been that everyone tries to encourage me with the old stand-by advice:

'Never give up'

Posted 4th June 2010

"Never give up" is a refrain I've heard every day since I had the stroke - sometimes multiple times in a day. Given that I don't really have a defeatist attitude, it makes me wonder how many times a day other [ones who are discouraged and/or depressed] stroke survivors hear it. It is apparently pervasive enough advice that Tedy Bruschi used it as the title of his book about his stroke recovery ...Loving him as I do, I have always understood that title to be the cheerleader in Bruschi encouraging other stroke survivors to keep plugging - that success will come. Like we're in a huddle together.

Every once in a while, though, I am tempted to give up - yesterday was a good example of a day when I spent a lot of time doubting that I would ever have my old life back. I don't mind hard work - in fact, I crave hard work, so that's not what's daunting. What's daunting is the endpoint - I don't want to work this hard and then fall short of my dream to have my former capabilities back. I know that the only guarantee is that if I don't do the work, I won't become more capable. So I am in a place where I have no choice but to continue putting my heart and soul into every day - but it's exhausting. I read an article in "Fast Times" yesterday about a research study that was done about self-control and it found that we can use up our self-control on one task and then not have it for a subsequent task. ... The study set-up was interesting because it put [two groups of] participants into [rooms] with one bowl of freshly baked cookies and [another] of radishes and told one group they could eat cookies and the other they could not. Afterward, the radish-eaters gave up on a task long before the cookie-eaters. I guess dieters should not expect to be able to tackle projects requiring persistence.

In [the movie] "Ever After," Prince Henry struggles with "caring," worried that if he starts caring about anything, there will be just too much to be concerned with and he'll be overwhelmed. I get that. The way my life is now, I have to be concerned about every little step - Is the ground even and stable? Is my weight distributed properly? Which leg goes first? Where to place my cane? Am I using the correct muscles in my left leg so that my leg doesn't swing to the side? Am I lifting my toe and landing heel first? Is my posture upright, with my midline centered, my left shoulder back? I'm sure I'm missing a few here, too. But each step gets analyzed in advance and then re-evaluated if something goes awry. So should I be expected to exhibit persistence in other projects in my life? Can't I just give up?

I know, I know: I am not supposed to give up because that's the only way to get my life back. No guarantees, though, just toil away in the void and hope that it makes the difference. Isn't that everyone's life, though? That makes me and my challenges really no different than anyone else.

Which gives me much more sympathy for other people, not just those with obvious troubles.

That blog entry merited this comment, from a stroke survivor named Dean Reinke:

Barb, I refer to it as braining my walking or driving or whatever. taken from another stroke forum person. She stated that she had to expend 100% of her brainpower into walking. This also applied to me at first, I couldn't walk and talk at the same time. Now if I use my cane I can walk and talk but without my cane I can talk only if I look down at the ground as I walk. Everything you are describing sounds familiar to most survivors and is helpful to getting currently enabled people to understand us. Dean

I think my optimistic post-stroke attitude has been fueled by letting the past define my goals, seeing the future brimming with possibilities I would never otherwise have achieved, and considering the present as the transition from one to the other. That leaves today full of hope and optimism.

Telling myself, "You can do it," is sometimes foolhardy and even incorrect, but the only downside is disappointment.

And remembering to tack "yet" onto the end of acknowledging a failure tosses more hope back onto my resources, as in, "I can't do it yet," replacing, "I can't do it."

Even pre-stroke I endured disappointments without catastrophe; I can do it post-stroke too. I knew that early on:

emotions

When I first had the stroke and the neurologists were explaining the repercussions it would have, one of them was the inability to hide my emotions, something that I did not find true: even though I was devastated, I managed to not once cry for myself while I was getting used to the idea; even though the stroke robbed me of my perfect life, my new circumstances were not so sad that I was inconsolable, I just had a new, dreadful challenge in my life. But I could bottle up my distress about it.

Of course, everyone told me to let out my negative emotions, and I've done it from time to time:

Pity party

Posted 22nd February 2010

I had a pity party today - something that I rarely do - and it happened while I was at therapy. It started, I think, because I've been very focused on getting my recalcitrant arm to work, which it hasn't, plus my shoulder has been bothering me so - it gets in the way of just about everything. Tom was supposed to be helping me with [shoulder] stretching exercises all week, but was unable to do them two days this week because my arm just hurt too much when we tried the exercises, which consist of making my arm bend in different positions in an attempt to stretch and loosen the muscles [primarily my pectorals]. I had been working with my OT trying to use the arm - she had me holding the back of a chair and tipping it toward me and then away without losing control of it, which actually went well - and then we went into a treatment room so that she could try to alleviate the pain or figure out what was causing it when we tried the stretching exercises. Lying there, with Tom standing by trying to re-enact our exercise failure, I found myself crying. Tom got me a tissue and my OT said, "Pain?" "No, I'm just feeling sorry for myself," I said. [She answered,]"You're entitled." Both she and Tom have the attitude that crying for myself is okay, that it's healthy and potentially helpful. I explained to them an enlightening concept that I'd read in Jill Bolte Taylor's book: Biochemically, our emotions hang around for only 90 seconds - if we're still feeling them (anger, fear, whatever) after that time is up, it's because we're choosing to keep that "circuitry" going, we're choosing to stay in that state. That means to me that a fleeting period of self-pity should be just that - fleeting; anything longer and I'm wallowing, something I will not do. Self-pity feels awful - helpless, hopeless and just downright painful - no way am I staying there. I'm choosing to feel good - and to feel good about myself at this point, I have to focus on progress - on what I can do now that I could not do a month or two or three ago. Or yesterday - that feels especially good - to be able to identify something that I just started doing today.

In PT today, I used the leg press for the first time and did 12 repetitions of I-don't-know-what weight, but it was hard and I suspect my quads might be sore tomorrow. That's a good thing.

Take note, though, that when I *do* cry, inevitably the person I'm with tries to get me to stop. Not overtly, like saying, "Don't cry, or "Suck it up." Rather, they hug me and/or tell me that things will get better, that I'm doing so well and I should be proud of myself, that they admire me and I'm an inspiration, all things that make me feel worse – under a microscope and as though I have to maintain my stoicism.

Why can't I be strong *and* cry? Why are my tears a problem that needs to be solved? Because they make my companion think less of me and he/she wants me back on that pedestal?

Cheerfulness

Posted Sept. 20, 2011

These days, it's hard being my husband or friend. Everyone, including my psychotherapist, encourages me to cry when I feel like it in order to release the emotion instead of bottling it up; yet, when I cry, these same people try to cheer me up - usually by reminding me of all of my blessings and suggesting that I be grateful for them. Well, you know what?!? I AM grateful for everything I have, but I'm grieving for everything I LOST. It's not rocket science. This morning I got frustrated in my attempt to don a camisole and asked Tom for help. Instead of doing what I asked - unrolling the back of it - he decided I should be putting it on a different way. Well, I was already frustrated because I had tried to do it by myself for too long before I asked for help, so I asked him - in a not-very-patient manner to please do what I had asked him to. (This falls into the same category of me asking him to get my blue coat from the closet and he brings the black one because he thinks it's more appropriate for the weather. Why can't I decide what coat I am going to wear? Am I 5 years old?) Then he got frustrated at the perceived criticism and snapped.

I certainly understand his frustration - and I know this life he has is not the life he wanted or planned for. I feel trapped enough for both of us, though, and part of that trap is the fact that those around me can express their emotions - sadness, disappointment and frustration - but as soon as I start, I am supposed to stop and put on a cheerful face.

No one, including me, wants me wallowing in self-pity, but the reality is that if I were to honestly express my emotions - as people encourage, but do not allow - I would cry all day every day. I know that would be an awful life - for me and for those around me - so I choose to go on good-naturedly and encourage others, letting them know that it's not unbearable after all.

One of the first things I did lying in my room in rehab was look into the past at the beautiful life I had built: there was nothing I wanted to fix back there. Back there I saw only things I had lost, things I used to do, things I had meant to do, and instantaneously I had to get used to having just a subset of that life, and I didn't get to pick and choose – I would get to do those things I was capable of, but had to leave behind those I could no longer do, no matter how much they meant to me. My body and brain would be determining what I got to do from now on. That was like waving a red cape in front of this bull ... I was *not* leaving my future out of my own control. I *would* again do the things I loved and had planned to continue doing indefinitely: rowing and my job, primarily; gardening was in there too. At first, getting back to my pre-stroke life was what I wanted. Over the years, that desire was whittled down to the gems: instead of managing at the newspaper, I would write; instead of gardening, I would enjoy what I could do in our yard. And instead of rowing, I *would row*. It was the only option there.

As I finally appreciated that writing was my profession and let go of working at the newspaper, and that there was a lot I could do in the yard using a new, better garden cart and hiring the teenagers up the street; I could finally focus on the future with the here-and-now as the starting location and the-best-I-could-do as an acceptable – and even desired – destination. One realization that helped, made a full *two years* following the stroke, was that helped was that life before was *not* perfect:

Idealizing the past

I ran into this by advice from M.K. Miller on Facebook:

If you're also starting over, remember: 1. RESIST THE URGE TO IDEALIZE WHERE YOU WERE.

She is not talking about idealizing a pre-stroke life, but I would like to ...

I have the tendency to relive the wonderful parts of my pre-stroke life - the productive workdays; laughing; my boss at his best; driving my Jetta on a beautiful day; coming in third in the Northeast Rowing Championship; running three miles to Good Harbor Beach, walking into the frigid water, then returning home to soak in our hot tub; moving things (dirt, mulch, water, plants, rocks and gravel) around in our gardens - without pasting in the negative parts. It's definitely an edited reality, revisionist history at its worst - because I truly believe THAT was my former life, and the pain of losing it is searing.

Having an airbrushed memory of the past prompts the unsolicited advice from others to not live in the past or in the future, but to focus on now - which I really don't want to hear because I am still very attached to the life I lost, working very hard now to return to it and having little clue what the future will deliver. To me, ignoring the past and the future to live "in the present moment" is a mistake: we learn from the past and plan for the future so that we are prepared for today's curve balls. I don't mean it's good to obsess about the past, worry about the future or waste the present. I would rather appreciate small pieces of the past and present and follow their trajectory into the future for me; that is the basis of hope.

Because of my relentless optimism, I tend to get my hopes up, which makes it hard to maintain that optimism when I fail to meet a goal. What I've learned though, is how to plow forward:

Keep on keeping on

Posted 27th January 2011

Lately, it's been challenging to be my most enthusiastic cheerleader; sure, I still have lots of people who love me and root for me, but I'm the one who most wants my recovery to happen, even on days that it seems unlikely, and I have to fire up my enthusiasm for working just as hard as I can every minute. As Dean [a blogging stroke survivor I quoted earlier], says, this is a 24/7 project.

Yesterday, my counselor suggested that I give myself an occasional break, during which I don't work on my recovery, but just indulge myself. My answer? "I can't." Taking a break and not working on recovery is just out of the question. Even as I sat there talking to her (and crying for the entire hour), I was trying to move my arm (unsuccessfully, let me add).

Sometimes I feel as though I'm about to have a breakthrough - I can feel the muscles I have to engage to move my arm/leg and I think I'm on the verge of actually doing it. Then I try and I fail. My body is teasing me, taunting me. Or is it my brain? Is my brain sick and tired of this, too? This scrutiny, the relentless demands?

That's it! Working on recovery is relentless - the despair, the repeated failures, the expectation that everyone has for me to be my buoyant can-do self, my continual disappointment in being trapped in this sub-par body with this sub-par mind.

I had one of those on-the-verge moments today: I was sitting near the wood stove, which was approaching the stage of needing wood and I was the only one around ...I was feeling as though my [affected] hand, with a fireproof glove, could pull up the top lid while my right hand loaded logs in the top, which is the usual loading door. I knew, I just knew that my arm could do it this time, but ...

As soon as I got my gloved hand under the handle to pull up on the lid, my arm failed me.[without catastrophe] ...

I don't know what it is that convinces me that THIS time my limbs are going to move properly, especially given that the feeling has not once been right. Not one single time out of something like 20 or 30. What's up with that?

Although my repeated goal has long been recovering my former life, my former capabilities, I eventually realized that I did NOT want ALL of my former life, just all of my former abilities. Even so, I could do without ever being able to run again. Where does that leave me? What is success recovery-wise?

Would it be okay to do my old tasks some new way, compensating for my lost abilities? Would it be enough to be able to carry a stack of dishes one-handed? Or would I need to use both hands, as I used to, to consider myself recovered? Two years post-stroke, I mused over the same issue:

recovering

Posted 3rd June 2011

What does "recovering from a stroke" mean? Do I have to fully return to my pre-stroke capabilities? Do I have to be able to use my left arm/hand to help me? Do I have to be able to run? Do I have to stop being so frustrated with my deficits? Must I be able to lie comfortably on my left side, the way I used to?

If I'm still limping, along with retaining other deficits two years from now, but have adapted to my life that way, am I recovered?

Or is recovered when I stop trying to move forward and just accept that how I am is how I will be?

Part of the difficulty in recovering is not knowing the endpoint. We are traveling on this exceptionally hard journey without knowing where we're going. We like to imagine where we're going - daydream about it, work even harder for our endpoint to be where we WANT it to be rather than what it's likely to be. We have abruptly lost control over half of our body [and much of our former lives], yet believe that we can control where we end up just through sheer pigheadedness, desire and hard work. We are an amazingly optimistic bunch. Encouraging, too - I have not once communicated with a stroke survivor who has not: patted me on the back, told me that I'm an inspiration or help to him/her, or told me a story about his/her own recovery that sheds light on my own struggle.

My Saebo unit [therapy for my arm and hand] should arrive here next week; the thought makes me dream of using my hand/arm again. For what? To carry things, to hug my family and friends, to help me with Turbo (brushing, petting and walking), to fold laundry, to open bags so that my right hand can put objects in, to help my other hand make dinner or plant things in the garden, to hold paper while I write on it, to stick my arm into clothing sleeves, to tread water, wring out a mop, hang clothes on the line... and the list is probably longer than that, but why are so many related to housework? I think it's because I love the prospect of doing every last thing I've been deprived of, appreciating the chance of doing even housework.

Maybe that's the definition of recovery: being able to clean my house. :)

That blog entry merited this reaction from another blogging stroke survivor (Linda Cooper, from Winnepeg):

"I have been having kind of a rotten day and was spending the better part of this afternoon crying.

"No real disaster.. just really overtired and stressed with my therapy and moderately annoyed with my physio guy today. I have only 4 more appts with my occupational therapist and today, Tony the physiotherapist, started talking to me about calling it quits with the physio soon. I am not sure what I am going to wind up doing next. I have an interview next week to get into a vocational rehabilitation program and I am actually very worried about it.

"I read your post and wow are you ever on topic for me again today.

"You said..."Part of the difficulty in recovering is not knowing the endpoint. We are traveling on this exceptionally hard journey without knowing where we're going. We like to imagine where we're going - daydream about it, work even harder for our endpoint to be where we WANT it to be rather than what it's likely to be.

"You said it so well. I think my daydreams are even confused right now."

"I was sitting there still blowing my nose and I read your housework comment and I just splurted out laughing so hard. Talk about keeping things in perspective! lol

"Recovery is being able to clean the house!!! ahhh one of those life long journeys."

All along, my stated ultimate goal has been to be able to row in a gig boat without help; my dream was to write this book *after* accomplishing that goal (Look at the title: "Stroke After Stroke").

Instead, I jumped the gun on putting the book together, assuming that I'd get back to being able to row by the time I completed the manuscript.

Looking back now, I see that the assumption that success was imminent has lured me since the beginning. After having the stroke one November, I planned to row the upcoming season (starting in spring) and even race by the following fall. At the end of each season since then I have expected to row the following one, and have set up step-wise goals through the off-season.

As each season starts, I keep on working hard in the hope that I'll be able to row without help by the end of *that* season. Ditto for this season – 2014 – which already started 4 months ago.

The year after I had the stroke, an Intel executive (Sean Maloney) had one. A kayaker, Maloney was told he "would never row again." The way I heard the story was that just after getting home from the rehab hospital, he insisted on going kayaking, and he went. Even though he could row only one-handed, which took him in circles, he considered it a success because he had just proven that his doctors were wrong about him never rowing again. I didn't know anything about Maloney until it made the news that he was miraculously returning to his job one year after the stroke. So in 2011, his success gave my faith in successfully returning to my job and rowing once more a shot in the arm. I was revved up again to believe I could do it. Again, I brazenly concluded that I would regain the use of my left arm/hand so that I could row, and, pigheadedly, that I could continue working for the newspaper.

Deciding to quit my editor job at the paper took me until the spring of 2013, when it became clear that the problems my job caused in my life were just flat-out not worth it: the positive aspects no longer outweighed the negative, and I resigned. One goal not met (keeping my job), but not because I failed and gave up. The reason was that I chose to eliminate it as a goal. I did not give up. I chose to walk away because I no longer wanted to do it.

I made a similar decision when I chose to stop using the Saebo when I made no progress after using it 2 hours per day for 7 months. I did not give up. I wisely chose to spend my time in a more productive way. I had better, more effective things to do.

But rowing? Having the goal of being able to return to an activity a survivor is passionate about is supposed to result in the best recovery outcome. For example, a golfer works hard on the skills required to be able to golf (walking on uneven ground, balance, grasping a club, etc.), more diligently than if his goal is to attach clothespins to pegs in a therapy room. I have no better way to recover than by diligently working toward rowing again.

156

Like Mahoney's first trip in his kayak, for me to row a gig boat again would be triumphant proof that my doctors and therapists were wrong. Being out there on the harbor - stretching forward, pulling back, working up a sweat, watching boats and the surface of the water as they pass, breathing salt air, laughing with my friends – there is no better way to spend my time, no more effective path to recovery – it's exactly the success I want.

Part of our recovery is to make our way through the quagmire of our emotions, to closely examine what we're doing, to tease the chaff of our misguided expectations from the tangle of our desires. To determine what we truly want, not automatically retain the assumptions about what we think we want. To live an examined life.

Why survive a potentially fatal event, only to fall back into the comfortable rut of your former life? Here is my unsolicited advice to anyone working on a recovery, based on my experiences:

1. Examine the details in your life, and revise your priorities if you don't like what you see. Train your magnifying glass on yourself, your relationships (friends and family), your profession, your particular job, and your way of life.

2. Then, be grateful for the positive things you find there. Eliminate the rest, without feeling pressure to justify yourself. You are not required to explain your desires. You have been given a second chance. Use it wisely.

Choosing an Attitude

Posted 11th February [2011]

Amy, of the mycerebellarstrokerecovery blog, recently wrote about becoming happy in her post-stroke life, about jettisoning those things/people who don't contribute to her happiness. That got me thinking: When the stroke struck me, I remained conscious throughout and was aware of the facts ER and MGH personnel communicated, but I never felt afraid. In addition to being quiet, unemotional and introspective, along with having slurred speech, I had an inability to focus on anything that mattered – like having had a stroke. For example, my dinner tray would arrive at my bedside in rehab and absorb all of my attention, distracting me from my family or whatever visitors I had. Friends might drive an hour or more to visit, wheel me into the hospital's sunroom, and then when we finished discussing one topic, I would turn my wheelchair around and start to leave the room. Someone – usually Tom - would tell me that I should stay because the visitors were not planning to leave yet, and then turn my chair around and push me back to the visitors, which I imagine now was awkward for everyone. But I was too zoned out to be aware of all things at once: the Zakim Bridge outside the sunroom windows, trying to not slump in my wheelchair, following the conversation, wondering how things were going at work, trying to get my hand to function, and hearing a woman crying out in garbled speech, etc. ....

In the first two days of my numbed, shell-shocked behavior, while educating himself about stroke, Tom stumbled along, trying to grasp what the repercussions of the stroke were. Out at dinner the other night, Tom told me that in those first two days, he wondered if he would spend the rest of his - mine, really – life caring for a me as an unresponsive and barely functioning [invalid] (but able to eat anything put in front of me), still overwhelmed by having life going on around me; and that scared the hell out of him. He admitted that, given how hard it's been dealing with me as I am (not that I think I'm anywhere near easy, but I'm pretty independent), he could not have done it if I'd been less capable. On the other hand, I think he'd have done fine – because sometimes you have no other choice than to suck it up and decide to make your life the best it can be.

Our daughter was 10 when she was diagnosed with Type 1 diabetes. She and I spent the first three days after her diagnosis in the hospital learning about diabetes management and proving we knew enough for the medical personnel to set her - a fragile fledgling bird - out into the world in my care. Every night in the hospital, I lay on a cot next to her bed, silently crying, on my back with tears running from the outside corners of my eyes into my ears. My running thought, like a hamster in a wheel, was, "This is not the way her life was supposed to be." I was angry and afraid, and thought my indignation was a reasonable response. She, though, was very pragmatic, keeping track of the number and locations of her many shots. She told me many years later that she thought she'd be treated for those three days in the hospital and then sent home cured; that sounds similar to my prognosis for a stroke – four weeks working hard in rehab, then home-free. Have I mentioned that I was numb and shell-shocked?

Only a few months after my daughter's diagnosis, once we had settled into [a] diabetes routine, I asked her how she could remain so cheerful, why she never got angry about having diabetes. Her answer? That she had two options: being sad or being happy, and why should she be miserable? In the time since the stroke, I have thought often of my wise and stoic 10-year-old. I admire stoicism for just two reasons: (1) it

159

prevents loved ones from experiencing even more pain and (2) it works to prevent being subsumed in the self-pity abyss. On the downside of stoicism, a study I once read supported the hypothesis that cancer patients who actively seek support from others end up living longer than those who depend on themselves to cope emotionally. What I saw as a remarkable aspect of my daughter's reaction was that she pushed disappointment off to the side and, instead of looking that way, she focused on what she truly wanted - happiness.

What if we all saw disaster as an opportunity to choose happiness?

Recovering your profession

The stroke has included completely re-defining my profession, something you may have to do also.

At the time I was struck, I had a job I loved more than any previous one in my 35-year work history. My boss made it clear that he was holding my job for me – both as managing editor and as general manager of the company.

It turned out though, that even though I was certain I could return to my position and do a good job there, I was too damaged cognitively to live up to our former standards; but because of my agnosia, I couldn't evaluate myself properly to know I was screwing up. I don't have sequential blog entries about disasters at work because I didn't feel as though I could spill my guts on my blog about messing up at work. That was a rule – no blogging about my job or co-workers.

Don't Do It!!

My first OT and my physiatrist both disapproved of me starting to work so soon after the stroke – about a month (Actually, I did some editing on my laptop while I was still in the rehab hospital. Ever since, I've wondered whether I did an adequate job.) The OT suggested not going even part-time for 3 months, while my physiatrist said 6 months. I, of course, knew better, and did exactly what I wanted: I started working as soon as I could read an entire e-mail message without Tom's help.

Perhaps that's why my re-entry was such a failure, and I started having to give up responsibilities, piece by piece.

That ability to recognize and appreciate my previous successes has helped me post-stroke – now doing anything for the first time is a reason to do a happy dance (in my heart, anyway, if not for real). This applies to both work and my physical recovery.

My yardstick has changed now - firsts now, as opposed to efficiency - but I still expect to continue advancing.

I have defined myself as a writer since I was a child. Along the way, that has included technical writing, newspaper reporting, a work-for-hire book about the history of Worcester, Mass., and four unpublished novels. As I was writing, I have always had another, wage-earning, job. Writing now, though, is my primary focus, my profession. For me, it brings the satisfaction my husband has always found in his work. For many years, he has said, "I can't believe they pay me for something I would do for free."

For a long time, both Tom and I have considered ourselves lucky that we have loved our jobs, given how others complain about theirs – the work, the hours, the demands, the stress – and how they look forward to Fridays. Tom and I have enjoyed weekends, but always looked forward to Mondays.

Toward the end of my second post-stroke summer, I attended a picnic for stroke survivors with aphasia – trouble with language. The symptoms range from people who have to relearn what all those squiggles on the paper are, to those who cast around in their heads searching for the correct words as they are speaking. Aphasia is generally the result of damage to the left side of the brain, which means that survivors who have hemiparesis on their right sides are those who often have language limitations.

Despite all the bad things that the stroke did to me, I appreciate something about the particular stroke I had - it was on the right side of my brain, so: (1) my language skills were left intact – except for slurred speech as the stroke was occurring - and (2) I lost the use of my non-dominant side instead of my dominant (i.e., I am right-handed and lost the use of my left side).

At the aphasia picnic, I met a woman who had spent the first years of her career as a Spanish teacher. Two months before having a stroke, Marian had been promoted to be the principal of an elementary school. I don't know how affected her language skills were, but at the picnic, her speech seemed fine to me. She had made the same mistake I did: she returned to her work as a principal too soon, and the job was beyond her. After failing as a principal, she was scheduled to return to teaching Spanish two weeks after the picnic. It was ironic, I think, for someone with aphasia to teach a language because it is easier for her to do than her previous job.

If/when you do return to work, if that's in your plan, expect to make mistakes.

Despite many frustrations caused by the limitations of the stroke, I am proud of myself that I did my best – inadequate as it was - at work, always giving my all and doing what I thought made the newspaper better. And I tried my hardest for three-and-a-half years post-stroke, not giving up, not resigning in frustration, but rather, resigning on good terms with my former boss. Combined, pre-stroke and post-, I spent more than 4 years as managing editor.

Not only was the stroke responsible for the loss of my job at the newspaper, it also gave me a career more true to myself and more suitable for my life and abilities – writing. Thank God.

In that way, although giving up my job was long, painful, and broke my heart, it was actually one of the best outcomes of having the stroke.

Although being unable to do your previous job might seem unbearable - Yes, I'm sure you're the only employee who can possibly do exactly what should be done, and no one could do better - your employer has been functioning fine without you while you were in the hospital/rehab.

Is there a way to look at your future seeing the end of that job as the beginning of following your heart's desire?

Working on reconstruction

Joann Murphey, a writer who is also a stroke survivor, has an old blog post about grief. In addition to the standard five stages of grief described by Kubler-Ross, Jo mentioned a stage called "Reconstruction."

I imagine the reconstruction phase as the one I'm in currently: trying to make something meaningful out of the rubble that resulted from the stroke. I'm working on creating a life in which I'm happy, productive, and moving forward.

After suggesting that your new life not include any negative aspects, I see that it's not always do-able: Now that you've jettisoned every negative thing from your life, what about those that are not that easy to get rid of? What if you can't work? What about having friends and relatives (and sometimes strangers) say hurtful things?

What about my own inability to row yet? Yes, I can keep working toward that goal, but it's still a huge negative (although perhaps trivial to others) aspect of my life. As are not being able to walk easily or use my hand. What about my feelings of grief? How do I jettison all that? Impossible, although I've tried.

Last February (2014), I realized I might be on the wrong track regarding eliminating the negatives as sound advice:

The End

[A] stroke survivor has been given a second chance and now has the opportunity to rebuild a life, to do a reset. I have suggested examining his/her life and keeping the positive components, while rejecting the negative ones. "Jettison the negative," is the common phrase. This includes rejecting friends and family members who are unsupportive or critical; eliminating negative thoughts and remaining positive; and recognizing blessings and expressing gratitude.

While those are good suggestions that might be a fine first step for survivors inundated by negativity and struggling to breathe, I actually don't believe it's a mature, self-aware response to pain. I don't find that a quest to reject everything negative from a life solves problems; instead it shuts a person down and guards against opportunities to grow.

And it's not what I've done in my own post-stroke life, so why [am] I giving that trite advice to others? Instead, my response has been to try to counter, rather than reject, the negative.

This pilgrimage of mine, my trek toward recovery, has encouraged me to meet frustration, anger, and insults with kindness, not my own anger and resultant rejection. To remain open and communicative, not shut down. It has worked for me – I am happy and well adjusted, although not complacent or accepting of my limitations.

Intermission IV: How to reach acceptance

Since becoming disabled by a stroke, I have rejected the concept of accepting my broken body the way it is – I have equated acceptance with giving up, and I am certainly not one to give up. In fact, the "Never give up" mantra is one I've heard scores of times, and I don't find it helpful. You know why? Because giving up is not one of the options on the menu in my head; so as advice, it goes in one ear and then nowhere. Seriously: Why would I accept my paralysis [correction: hemiparesis, muscle weakness, actually] and give up trying to overcome it? How could I? And how could I ever accept the fact that I could be disabled the rest of my life, a timespan that might be 40 [no way: I'm 56 now, so 30 is more likely] more years ... Can I really accept being like this for 40 years?

One OT I've had along the way once told me about a conversation she'd had with a patient who had broken her arm in four places; she asked the OT when her arm would be back to normal. The OT's response? She told the young woman that her arm would never be the same again – that it would always be an arm that had been broken in four places; what COULD happen, though, was that she could regain all the functions her never-broken arm had been able to do.

And this struck me the other day: What if acceptance means that I can stop going into the rattrap of focusing so far into the future? What if it means that I continue my fight, my hard work, never knowing the endpoint, never knowing how long it will last? Yes, I know where I want to go. Surprisingly, it is NOT back to where I was. I imagine a new, improved Barb, someone with all the physical and mental capabilities as pre-stroke, but with a deeper understanding of people in pain, grieving and/or taking a shot at the "impossible," a writer better able to pierce the hearts of my readers by shining a light on situations they assume they will never find themselves in. I plan to be wiser, more empathetic, encouraging and connected to others.

There is no getting around the fact that I will always be a woman who has had a stroke. I can accept that.

My future

In our quest for recovery, desperation takes stroke survivors on many tangential paths. I have tried nearly every healing method I've heard about, including the Eastern practices of Kundalini Yoga (I have tried practicing both Kirtan Kriya briefly and Breath of Fire intermittently), Tong Ren healing (my take: rhythmically bashing a rubber doll on different places depending on the injury), sound therapy (the practitioner analyzed my speaking voice to identify the tones I was missing and the muscles correlated with each, then gave me a recording of those missing tones for me to listen to for hours each day), Christian laying-on-of-hands healing and prayer, and chanting the Buddhist "nam-myo-ho-renge-kyo" for 15-minute daily sessions.

Then there are the procedures at the edge of medical acceptance: craniosacral therapy, acupuncture (for me, needles into the appropriate spots in the homunculus that is my ear), and meditation.

In addition to all of that, I have spent countless hours doing traditional prescribed exercises, walking, using Nautilus equipment, rowing on my Concept II, using my eStim, doing mirror therapy, using a Saebo, and doing aquatic therapy.

And I go to a psychotherapist to help me with my grief, which is still present nearly 5 years post-stroke.

The components of my new life (my new normal) must include an appreciation of life, independent of circumstances. I will never be happy *about* my current physical state, but I'm working on happiness *despite* it. Secondly, for me to feel productive includes two components: creating meaningful professional work (as a writer) and helping and encouraging others.

There has been nothing that has sustained me more during this pilgrimage than the encouragement I've received from family, friends, and even strangers. It's important to me to radiate that support and encouragement to others. That means exhibiting love and concern at all times, including in the face of negativity. As stroke survivor Jim Sparks once wrote, one challenge in life is to not become negative in the face of negativity.

The third facet (moving forward) means plugging on with my therapy and celebrating the improvements I experience. Even if I don't reach my goals before I die, I will still be working on my recovery when I do. I will not give up.

It took me 52 years to create the perfect life I had before having a stroke. I have from now until the end of my life to create my second life, and I mean for it to be just as happy, productive and enjoyable as my previous one. Yes, it will be a life very different from what I had before, very different from what I would be living had I not become disabled by having a stroke, or if I had already recovered from the stroke.

There it is, the story of my trek following a stroke, my journey since losing control over half my body, while I pursue my goal of once again rowing in Gloucester Harbor.

Four years and seven months later, I still haven't reached my destination. Not yet.

But I will not lose heart or determination.

As I have been on my pilgrimage, persistence and patience have been my two constant friends. Like you – and everyone else, even those who have not lived through tragedy - I don't know what the future holds, except that I will pursue my goal of rowing once again.

Recovery, like rowing, is propelled by tireless hard work, relentless repetition, and small increments of progress. To paraphrase E. B. White (in *Charlotte's Web*), it might take the rest of my life to accomplish my goal, but that's what I have.

Please take comfort in the fact that (as Peter Levine has written), your recovery will be the hardest thing you ever do.

Barbara Polan
Bayberry Ledge
July 2014

Acknowledgements

I would most likely not be alive without my husband, Tom, who identified my stroke and prevented me from driving to work the morning that my symptoms started showing themselves.

In addition, he and my four siblings were my caregivers for my first 6 weeks at home. For my siblings' rotation as they passed the responsibility for me from one to another, relieving Tom of the burden, I owe them all more than I can say.

As for this manuscript itself, I have to thank my first readers – Kathy, Trisha, Maureen and Nancy - all of whom gave me constructive criticism that helped me vastly improve how I told my story. Special thanks to Kathy for her detail-oriented editing. Despite their contributions, any mistakes or tedium in this edition are all mine.

And there is no group I appreciate more than the Gloucester Gig Rowers for their encouragement throughout my ordeal as I try – and try again – to row.

Cover design by Emily Ianacone:
www.myfriendemily.com

Cover photo courtesy of the Gloucester Gig Rowers.